# AN HONEST LOOK
# AT A MYSTERIOUS JOURNEY

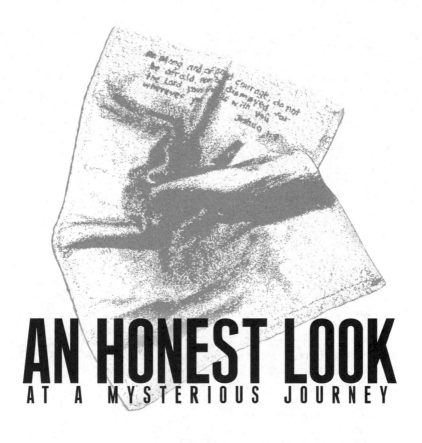

# AN HONEST LOOK

## AT A MYSTERIOUS JOURNEY

## JOHN & JOANNA STUMBO

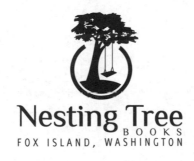

## Nesting Tree

BOOKS

FOX ISLAND, WASHINGTON

Cover Design: Jeff Brown, Salem, OR
Interior Design: Deborah Schermerhorn, Colorado Springs, CO
Editor: Elizabeth Honeycutt, Glendale, AZ
Back Cover Photo: Jenn Whiteman, Colorado Springs, CO

Published by Nesting Tree Books
655 6th Avenue
Fox Island, WA 98333

Printed in the United States of America.

ISBN:  978-0-9839333-0-4

*To all those who have*
*run*
*walked*
*stood*
*sat*
*or*
*knelt*
*with us on this journey*

"You listen to a testimony like John Stumbo's and you cry because there are many things we will never understand. But we wipe away the tears because we know how a Sovereign God is able to even take the weak of this world to tell a story that will confound the wise. This is one of the most powerful stories that I have ever heard. It will change the way you face life's twists and turns."

*Ravi Zacharias, author and speaker*

# CONTENTS

# PART TWO

# PART THREE

# AUTHORS' EXPLANATION

"It's your book!" Joanna does not like the suggestion that her name appear on the cover as co-author.

"But, it's *our* story." I think it is a great idea to have Joanna's name appear on the cover as the co-author.

I try to strengthen my case, "Besides you did write some of it."

"Just a few chapters." This is not the first time in our marriage that Joanna downplays her own contribution.

"I should have had you write more."

"No. It's your book."

"But, it's our story."

And, we're back to where we started.

In all fairness to Joanna, I did back her into this project. I never once said, "Let's write a book together." But a few dozen pages into my writing, I discovered that I needed her help more than I first realized. This is not the first time in our marriage that I've committed to a project and then realized that I needed to drag Joanna into it. Joanna was reluctant at first, but she understood my dilemma.

I appealed, "I wasn't even conscious for five days of the story. You gotta help me. I can't tell that part of the story with the accuracy and emotion that you can."

She consented. I liked what she wrote and found a few excuses for her to write more. Meanwhile, we spent tens of hours recalling the many experiences that this book chronicles. More than once we said to each other, "I didn't know that's what you were feeling at the time."

So the writing of this book truly has been a team project and "Team Stumbo" is the better for having written it together. The majority of what you are about to read are John's words, but Joanna has been consulted on them all. The chapters that Joanna has written are clearly identified.

I gloat that Joanna's name is on the cover, "For once I won an argument!"

"It's your book, so the final decision is yours." Joanna's words have that "conversation over" tone to them.

"Wait. Huh? So did I really win the argument?"

———— ✺ ————

One more note of explanation: you may be wondering about the front cover graphic. To some it looks like a wadded up piece of paper. There have been plenty of those in the writing of this book. But, the graphic isn't crinkled paper. Another person assumed it was an old map...like a treasure map. If we could have found a map to guide us through this "mysterious journey" we certainly would have treasured it. However, there was no map.

The graphic on the cover is of a spit rag...one of my very own. Yes, this may be the world's only book with a spit rag on the cover. You'll understand the graphic's significance as you read.

So, welcome to our world. Welcome to the story we never intended to write...or live. As the title indicates, we've promised "an honest look." We'll do our best to deliver on that promise.

# PREFACE
## THE LOVE AND HATE OF RETELLING THE STORY

I'm stalling. I admit it.

Month after silent month has passed. Excuses have multiplied. Life's happened.

I know the day will come when I will record the story of my sudden illness and long recovery, but I'm dragging my feet.

Meanwhile, people are telling me: "Just compile your blogs and make them into a book."

It's a great idea. I'll eventually pursue it. But the blogs, important though they are, don't tell the full story. The blogs are devotional reflections and focused snapshots of a portion of my journey, but I've sensed that I need to make the "movie" version—to start the story at the beginning and let it run uninterrupted.

I privately wonder, *Why can't I get started? I will write my story someday. I must write it. What holds me back?*

I know I need to set aside large blocks of time—entire days, many days—and allow my mind to reenter the hospital rooms, rehab centers, and the living room chair where I spent so many months. Yet, I must do more than that. I must allow my mind to reenter all that those places represent: mystery, pain, fear, peace, loss, hope, crisis, depression, laughter, tears, questions, prayers, hallucinations, kindness, gloom, tenderness, abandonment, perseverance, healing, and grace.

It occurs to me that I have stumbled upon the key reason for my hesitation: To write a story is to experience it again. A story must be relived to be recorded.

Something within me recoils: *Why would you want to go through all of that again?*

Yet something else beckons me on: *Others will benefit from your story. Write!*

And so, I begin.

As I write, I discover how equally enjoyable and difficult the writing process can be. Some moments bring great pleasure—I find fulfillment in crafting sentences, recreating scenes, and retelling the story. Other moments deliver darker emotions. The human soul resists dredging up all the silt that has settled, but it has an amazing capacity to relive the experiences once forced to do so.

The human mind, it seems, isn't the only part of us that has memory—our emotions do as well.

Yet, as I proceed, it seems that the act of writing assists my own healing process. I pray that the reading of it will assist you as well.

Above all, I want God to be glorified. Every story must be about Him in the end. No story truly ends with us. All streams of existence originate from Him and ultimately flow to Him.

———— ∞ ————

My wife, Joanna, walks by and flips on a light. I have been unaware that nightfall has wrapped the room in its darkness. The light from my laptop screen has been sufficient for me to continue to type. I've become unaware of my surroundings for so long that I sit alone in the darkness… and I write on.

I write, knowing that thousands of you have walked this journey with me and, in a sense, deserve to know more of the story. By offering an inside look at my thoughts and experiences, perhaps you will now know why God laid my story so heavily on your heart. I'm referring to people who have wept for me, fasted from food for me, been awakened in the middle of the night and prayed for me, started every Thursday morning with me as they read my weekly blog post, started every meal for over a year praying that I would someday be able to eat as well, started every jog with a prayer that I'd someday resume running, worked in my yard when my legs were too unsteady to even walk in it, experienced genuine grief over my loss and true joy in my healing.

In the most practical and profound ways, you have fulfilled the scriptural command: "Rejoice with those who rejoice; mourn with those who mourn" (Romans 12:15).

I sense that I owe you this retelling.

Your life and mine are interwoven—our stories intermingle—and so as I retell my story, perhaps your story will come more clearly into focus or have more meaning. Perhaps the insight I've received will help you gain fresh perspective.

What is more, I've become increasingly aware that the potential benefit of this story is not limited to those individuals who have journeyed this trail with me. At first, I assumed that my story of physical illness would touch others who struggle with health issues. What I underestimated is just how adaptable the human story can be.

People with issues far different from mine are finding that we share similar emotions and benefit from similar lessons. Change the scenario slightly from physical to financial issues, for example, and our souls still find a connection. Human pain—whether it comes in the form of broken bodies, broken relationships, broken hearts, or broke bank accounts—has a great deal in common.

And so I write. I write for my own healing. I write for those who've journeyed with me. I write for those I have never met but who will find slices of their own story in these pages. I write for God because it seems that He kept me alive to do just this.

Grace and peace to you as you read.

# PART ONE

I know, O LORD,
that a man's life is not his own;
it is not for man to direct his steps.

*Jeremiah 10:23*

# JOGGING TRAILS, WALKING PEWS

It was one of those October days when summer seemed reluctant to say "goodbye" for another year, and I was reluctant to bid it farewell.

October 18, 2008, was a good day from the start. The forested trails of a local park provided the setting for a small group of my jogging friends to talk, laugh, sweat, and enjoy being alive together. After my friends left, I lingered at the park to run a little farther and make it a ten mile morning.

I'm glad that I didn't know that the next time I would visit this trail I would be in a wheelchair. Ignorance of our future is a form of God's grace. Few of us would be able to fully embrace today if we knew what tomorrow held. My day would have been spoiled had I known what was before me.

But I didn't know. And I enjoyed. The air smells better, food tastes richer, and life feels more "alive" when a person is in good enough shape to painlessly appreciate a long run. To be able to do these things with people you love triples the pleasure.

My jog completed, I stopped by the local YMCA to finish my workout by lifting a few weights. A warm shower, a good lunch, and an hour relaxing at home provided the bridge I needed to mentally shift into gear for what the rest of the day held.

It was Saturday. In a few hours, nearly a thousand people would gather at Salem Alliance Church for the first of our weekend services to worship and receive a message from the Bible. My sermon was complete, but I wasn't quite ready to preach it. First, I needed to prepare myself.

The cheerful sounds of the worship team's rehearsal greeted me as I opened the church doors. Tech team members busily adjusted lights, video cameras, and microphones. The janitorial crew ensured that the building called the "church" was ready for the people called the "church" to arrive. I grabbed my Bible and sermon notes from my office and stepped into the back row of the 1,200 seat auditorium.

I don't know when the habit first started, but I find that before I preach, I like to "walk the pews." As the worship team's music filled the room, I added my prayers row-by-row. Slowly zigzagging my way from back to front, I prayed through my message, prayed for those who would sit in the seats I was passing through, and prayed for my own heart. It was my simple effort to prepare for the services to follow.

On this weekend, it was my privilege to launch a new series on the *Names of God*. Recent economic upheaval in America had prompted our pastoral team to ground our messages in something solid and unchangeable. In our planning meetings, we reasoned, "What is more solid and unchangeable than the character of God? And what better way to talk about His character than through the names that He bears?"

As I prepared for the series, I ran across a statement from author Timothy Stoner who described God as being "untamed, unfathomable, unpredictable, yet utterly and infinitely good."

In the column of my sermon notes, I scribbled a broken sentence revealing my response to this God I could not adequately describe, "Yielding myself into the hands of the Confusing One who rarely gives explanations and seeing it as an exhilarating adventure."

Little did I know the significance of those words for my own life. Little did I know just what kind of adventure awaited me.

This sermon would be the last one I would deliver for months, and I would not preach regularly again for almost two years, at least not from a pulpit. To my great surprise, a "congregation" did gather around a blog I would write in my recovery. My "sermons" for the season took the form of rants and reflections that found their way from my keyboard to cyberspace. This "congregation" would bless me countless times and pray innumerable prayers.

But for now, I knew none of this.

It had been a good day. I would do my best to make it a good night as well. And so as I walked the pews, I prayed to this One whom I believe to be the epitome and the source of all goodness.

The adventure was about to begin.

# DAY 2

"Did you switch brands of laundry detergent again?"

I discovered a mild rash under my clothing and figured it must be my wife's fault...which says more about me than I care to admit. Years ago, Joanna washed our clothes with a type of detergent that had given me a rash, but since then she had faithfully purchased a more expensive product on my behalf.

Joanna assured me that she hadn't made any product changes, and I responded to the symptom as I normally do: I ignored it. However, I was soon dealing with a second symptom: a flu-like "bleh."

I'm quite sure that "bleh" isn't a word you'll find in a medical dictionary, but I'm also quite sure you know the feeling. You're not very sick yet, but something has snuck in and is siphoning off your energy. Somewhere mysteriously within you, the tide is going out and taking your sparkle and zip with it.

This case of the "bleh" wasn't bad enough to steal my enthusiasm for the day. The weekend services at church were uplifting. Salem Alliance has a well-earned reputation for being an encouraging place to attend and serve. I knew I was a blessed man to lead such a healthy church.

But this weekend was especially significant. For two decades, our church leaders prayed for and tried to acquire a half-block of land adjacent to our property. In recent years, we had finally been able to purchase the parcel—which by then was two defunct used car sales lots—

and, after countless meetings, we were now ready to move ahead with a major construction project.

I led the Sunday afternoon congregational meeting where affirmation for the new project was strong. It made me genuinely happy to sense the spirit of unity and faith among us. The new building we were designing—"a convergence of community, church and commerce"—would be a faith-stretching, city-impacting project. I knew that many churches would not have had the vision to pursue it. Yet, before me sat an assembly of church members who were willing to believe and build.

Today Broadway Commons, with its free medical clinic, coffee shop, conference rooms, leased office spaces, amphitheater, and dedicated prayer center, beautifully adorns the landscape and lifestyle of the neighborhood. Yet, on this pleasant October afternoon, it was still just a parking lot and a dream.

I closed the meeting with a sense of fulfillment in my heart. The church was moving ahead. Not only were we just a few months away from groundbreaking for the new building, we were also fully staffed with a solid team. I breathed a prayer of relieved gratitude. The last year had not been easy as we navigated our way through a very difficult staff transition. Now we were moving forward in unity. Everything was good, except for this flu I seemed to be getting.

However, there was no time in my schedule for getting sick. I came home from the meeting to spend a few hours with my family and to pack. A family from our church graciously offered me their home on the Oregon Coast to use for a study break. I was eager to get there before it was too late in the evening so I could have a fresh start in the morning.

I gave Joanna and our son, Drew, hugs and threw two boxes of books, a cooler of food and a small suitcase into the trunk of our Saturn. The hour drive from our home to the Coast is scenic and often busy in the daylight, but on this night I enjoyed the tranquility of the quiet roads and peaceful evening.

I was a blessed man. I had a great wife, kids, church, and future. Oh, our marriage wasn't at a real strong point, but we had come through tough seasons before; we'd figure this one out as well. Maybe a week apart would do us some good.

For now, my bigger concern was to make significant progress on my doctoral dissertation. Maybe I'd get a chance to work on a book idea as well. Certainly I'd find time to enjoy a few good runs along the coast. I was really looking forward to these days.

Following the directions provided, I found my way down a narrow road running right along ocean front property. I spotted the house number, rolled the Saturn into the driveway, and was stunned by the beauty of the home. Salty air and the sound of crashing waves greeted me. This would be a good week.

I unpacked the cooler into the refrigerator, laid my books out on the large dining room table—wrapped by full length windows—and stared out at the thundering waves. I had everything I needed for a great week of dissertation writing: ample resources, an incredible view, and complete solitude. Grateful for my many blessings, I called it a night.

The "flu" symptoms hadn't subsided, but I'd be fine. I had no expectations on me for the next six days but to write in solitude. If I had to be sick somewhere, this was the perfect place.

# DAYS 3 THROUGH 8

*I look like Popeye,* I thought as I looked at myself in the bathroom mirror.

During the night my arms had swollen considerably. They looked large enough to be intimidating, but the fact was they were so weak I could barely lift them to brush my teeth. I was grateful that I had carried in my boxes of books from the car the night before because now I doubted I could lift them.

Happily, the "bleh" hadn't worsened and I ate a small breakfast while spending some time reading scripture and praying. It took me a few hours to get my mind fully engaged in my studies, but soon I was elbow deep into my research. Outlines began to form, schedules were made, and a few pages of text found their way into my laptop. I took a few short breaks to breathe the ocean air or check in with the office, but I was a man on a mission and I wasn't going to be deterred.

From morning to well into the evening I wrote. Monday flowed into Friday and my dissertation was being birthed. The Saturn sat ignored all week—I had all the food and resources I needed and was happy being alone. The television sat in silence—the music on my iPod and view from my window provided better entertainment. My running shoes sat motionless. Normally I would have run at least twenty-five miles during a week like this, but my body kept telling me this would not be a good idea. In fact, by late in the week the muscle weakness was settling into my legs as well. I could barely climb the stairs or walk a few blocks.

*I've never had a flu bug quite like this before.*

Yet, I wasn't worried. Why should I be? I was as healthy as any forty-seven-year-old I knew. I had never spent a day in the hospital since the week of my birth. I had great genetics: my father was strong and energetic until a car accident suddenly ended his earthly life at age seventy, my mom was independent and vibrant at eighty-nine, and my five siblings were all alive and well. I had healthy habits (especially if ice cream is considered an essential food group). I kept my weight down, avoided tobacco and alcohol, and had annual medical check-ups which only confirmed my good health. In recent years I even started running ultra-marathons.

Long distance running was something I hadn't envisioned for myself. I stumbled onto the pleasure of it quite by accident when, seven years earlier, we moved to the Willamette Valley with its pleasant parks and trails. Our daughter, Anna, was sixteen at the time and had taken up the hobby of jogging. I saw this as a perfect combination: an hour alone with my daughter on a beautiful trail every Saturday morning. What more could a dad want...even if it did require putting running shoes on my aging body and pounding out a few miles?

I had never been much of a runner. During my college years I mocked the cross country team. Why would anyone want to run the miles those athletes did when there was no ball involved? When I did run, it was only to get in shape for a real sport like basketball. I hated the sprints and line drills our coaches required of us. Running was a necessary evil, not a sport in and of itself.

As I grew older, however, I found myself making friends with the idea of running...if for no other reason than to keep my weight down. I like to eat and so a three mile jog was all the justification my mind needed for helping myself to a second dessert.

The pleasure I found in our Saturday jogs through the park caught me off guard. I loved the trees, rabbits, river, changing seasons, smell of the air, blackberries, birds, falling leaves, and the trail itself. I was overjoyed to get to spend these sweet moments with my daughter. I was delighted to discover that side-by-side we had conversations we may never have had face-to-face. To this day, these hours on the trail with my daughter are some of the happiest memories of my life.

Meanwhile, I was surprised to discover that I was developing a love of running. I felt alive and at peace on the trail.

Every Saturday, being the competitive creatures we are, Anna and I would push ourselves just a little further in the park. Three miles soon became four and then six. One day I realized that we were running half the distance of a half-marathon.

"Hey," I said to her after one jog, "If we keep this up we could do a half-marathon together sometime. What do you think?"

She instantly owned the idea and on a drippy January day, Anna and I ran our first race—she, winning her age division and I, plodding in quite a few minutes behind her. In the years that followed Anna would go on to become an eight-time All-American runner for her college in track and cross-country. She also became the women's marathon national champion for the National Association of Intercollegiate Athletics.

Meanwhile, I was still plodding along, running numerous half-marathons (13.1 miles), marathons (26.2 miles) and ultra-marathons (trail runs of thirty-one or more miles). I eventually qualified for the Boston Marathon and in 2008 I made the top ten list for ultra-marathon runners of my age division in Oregon. There were only a couple dozen of us my age crazy enough to run these races, but nevertheless it gave me the feeling of being alive and being strong. The unthinkable had happened: I had fallen in love with running.

One of my favorite things to do on a day off was to find a lonely trail and run fifteen or twenty miles. I know that this kind of running sounds odd or completely nuts to many people. A friend of mine teased, "You can get counseling for that, you know!"

But running was now my favorite pastime. I couldn't say with Eric Liddell, "God made me fast," but I could happily join him on the second half of his famous words, "When I run, I feel His pleasure."

But not this week. I'd have to let this mysterious "flu" run its course before I could run again. By Saturday I was encouraged by my writing progress but called Joanna with a problem.

"I'm not sure I can drive home," I confessed.

Something like this had never happened to me. The words felt strange coming out of my mouth. My head argued, *Of course you can drive. You are always the one who drives.* But from somewhere deeper I accepted her offer to bring Drew and come to get me.

It turned out to be a great decision.

# DAYS 9 THROUGH 24

Strength was being sapped from my muscles by the day. Upon returning home, I scheduled the first doctor's appointment I could. In the initial exam I heard the medical staff use words I couldn't believe I was hearing: disease words, life-altering words, names-of-conditions-that-I-knew-other-people-had-but-not-healthy-people-like-me words. What precipice had I just fallen off that a healthy guy like me was having a conversation like this?

I was sent to another doctor and more tests were run. By now the rash that I had once blamed on my wife had manifested itself in numerous places, most notably on my face. I looked like I wore a raccoon mask with inflamed cheeks and white eyes. Previously, I had the misconception that rashes were limited to things like irritated responses to chemicals or natural substances like poison ivy. I didn't know that the skin might send out warning flares announcing that something was seriously wrong inside the body.

Soon, sores stormed my mouth. It seemed that whatever was attacking my body began flaring up everywhere. My inner cheeks, gums, and tongue looked like a miniature minefield.

Next, my digestive and urinary system started to go haywire. Loss of appetite, agonizing constipation and a growing concern about my kidneys took my "bleh" to new depths. Meanwhile, blood tests revealed that my muscle enzymes were going crazy, registering many times higher than that of a normal person.

In the midst of this downward spiral, my doctor, wife, and I agreed that I should be hospitalized. There they could monitor my condition and be more aggressive at running tests. Immediately a sense of relief came over Joanna and me. I was submitting myself into the care of professionals and every decision wouldn't be up to us to make.

I wasn't pleased about the fact that they asked me to sign an authorization allowing them to cut open my left thigh, remove a small piece of my muscle, and stitch me back up. I'm convinced that the day will come when medical advances reach the point when some of our current practices, such as muscle biopsies, will be viewed as barbaric. But, I tried my best to be a cooperative patient and became extremely impressed by the compassionate concern and quality care I received from the Salem Hospital team. My first introduction to hospital living was a positive one. I even liked the food.

My body was a mess, but my spirits were still good. Friends came to visit and pray. I enjoyed getting to know the hospital staff. I had confidence that the doctors would figure out what was wrong and have some remedy or God would heal me or I would just get better—because, after all, I'm a healthy guy, remember?

The only real complaint I had about my hospital stay was that I found it a horrible place to get any sleep. This problem was compounded one night by the fact that I was now starting to struggle with significant pain. Up to this point I had felt very ill, but illness and pain are two very different things.

At 2:00 on a Friday morning, I called the church office knowing full well that no one was there. I made my way through the voice mail system to my executive assistant's desk. Kathy Bletscher had been an amazing support to me during my years of being lead pastor, but her servant heart only kicked into a higher gear once I became ill. She found ways to encourage and support me far beyond what the church paid her for or I could expect from her. I knew she would be happy to do a little dictation off her voice mail. A sermon was forming in my heart and I had to get it out. I fully expected to be back in the pulpit soon and thought I'd get a head start on a future message.

I was wrong. It was a sermon that wouldn't be preached…at least not until much later when its truths had been taken layers deeper in my heart. But on this night, as I had to keep redialing the Salem Alliance number because my sermon was far longer than the voice mail limits allow, this is a portion of what I "preached."

*I am sitting up in a chair with a bag of ice on each leg and am unable to sleep tonight due to severe muscle pain caused by an attack on my muscles. Various pain medications have been ineffective, and I am unable to lie in bed. I ask the aide to play the recording of last week's message from Salem Alliance, and I listen with great appreciation as our preaching team effectively continues our series on the Names of God speaking of Jehovah-Rophe, our Healer.*

*As I listen, I reach out with my swollen arms and welcome any healing that God might provide. I receive nothing in immediate response, but am reminded of the verse that I heard earlier today from Psalm 139 that celebrates that He is the God of the light and the darkness. Both belong to Him—both are His territory, both are His domain, both are His Kingdom, both are under His rule.*

*My left arm is connected to an IV continually feeding me fluids to protect my kidneys. My throat is like sandpaper because of the ban on any food or liquids until morning. My heart is encouraged by the biblical, firm, clear message—historic to the Christian faith—the message of a Healing Christ. I believe the truth of these words, even though I'm not yet experiencing them in my own body.*

*I find not from myself, but from a different Source, the confidence that God is good, He is in control, He is wise, He is all-knowing; He has bigger plans than the ways of man and His paths are good. And while I don't have an explanation, I have been given tonight in some ways a more powerful gift—a gift of trust and confidence that God is somehow involved in the darkness—the darkness of the room at this moment, the darkness of my condition at this moment—but a God who is involved and good. And He can only be good.*

*A peace that surpasses understanding; a peace that I don't really comprehend, guards my heart and mind in Christ Jesus. I don't have any sense that I am concocting this on my own; I feel it is a gift from Him that I have this sense of peace and trust of His goodness at this time, completely unaware of where it will lead in the months or years to come. I believe healing could come in an instant, or I have the strong possibility of having a condition for a lifetime. I don't pretend that there is no fear involved, but I rejoice in the fact that greater is He that is in me than the circumstance around me. This is an act of God's kindness, an act of healing of a different nature.*

*Whenever our fears are addressed by the kindness of God, that is a form of healing that might not be our first choice, but can become one of great power....*

I look back on that night with sweet memories. Physically I was experiencing some of the most significant pain I've known, but spiritually I was being protected and carried to new places. I wasn't getting any answers medically, but I had something more significant: hope.

After a week in the hospital, my condition seemed to stabilize and the doctors weren't really sure what to do next, so I was allowed to return home. A couple friends suggested that I really ought to go to a larger hospital like the respected Oregon Health and Science University (OHSU), but that seemed like a lot of hassle to me. I had a few prescriptions to take, I'd be careful to get plenty of rest at home, and I'd be fine. After all, I'm a healthy guy, right?

# DAYS 25 THROUGH 31

At first glance, the words "confidence," "naïvety," and "pride" may not have much in common. But it occurs to me in real life, the boundary lines between the words easily blur together. One can subtly and swiftly slip into the territory of another.

Confidence is often a positive characteristic of leaders. Because of it, we are able to move with expectancy into the future, make decisions and rally others to join us. I don't remember choosing or necessarily even wanting to be a leader, but from grade school through adulthood, leadership opportunities have been granted to me. I'm not sure what others saw in me, but my guess is that one thing they observed was confidence. I could be plagued with insecurity in certain situations, but when the right factors came together, I could move forward confidently.

Looking back, however, I have to admit that much of my confidence was based on naïvety. I was too clueless to know how big the obstacle was, so I just kept moving forward. The opinions of naysayers and realists—often wise and well-meaning—seemed to fall on deaf ears: mine. Was I truly confident or just dumb? Perhaps both!

Meanwhile, pride has to be included in the conversation. At times I was confident because, frankly, I thought I was better than my opponents or others around me. What may have appeared as confidence may have more accurately been skillfully cloaked arrogance.

As I left the hospital, a doctor explained to me, "If you had a common issue like a gall bladder problem or heart attack, we could tell you what we would do to take care of it, how long it would take and what your future prognosis would be. But since we don't know what you have, we aren't sure how to treat you, how long it will take, or what to expect for the future."

I appreciated his honesty, dodged his suggestion to go to OHSU, and returned home where I attempted to resume my work for the church. Looking back, I have to ask myself why I was reluctant to see the severity of my situation and be more proactive in pursuing solid answers. Was I *confident* that God was accomplishing something in my life or *naïve* about how serious my situation was or *proud* of my good health and habits? My answer: all of the above as the lines aren't distinct.

In my own defense, I would argue that I like living this way. I like the approach that David took in the twenty third Psalm. He wasn't a glass-half-empty or a glass-half-full kind of person. He was a glass-running-over kind of person, "You prepare a table before me in the presence of my enemies...my cup overflows" (Psalm 23:5).

Much of the ministry at Salem Alliance is set up on the basis of teams. The Pastoral Management Team makes many of the day-to-day decisions impacting the church. The Preaching Team crafts sermon series together and takes turns preparing and presenting the messages to the congregation. The Governing Board meets weekly and enjoys genuine fellowship with each other.

These, and many other church teams, continued to serve well in my absence. Unlike many churches that are heavily dependent upon one person, the leadership and responsibilities at Salem Alliance were well disseminated. I'll confess that as the lead pastor this arrangement was awkward for me at times, but when my illness struck, our church structure served us well.

I kept in regular communication with the church office while in the hospital, but now that I was home, I wanted to be all the more engaged. Kathy, my assistant, brought me my correspondence, consulted me on issues, and took dictation for various communications I wanted to get from my head onto paper. Important decisions were being made about the new building design and plans were forming for our Thanksgiving and Christmas services. I didn't want to miss out on any of these preparations. Why should a little sickness stop me from staying fully engaged with the church I love?

The pain throughout my muscles had lessened, my mouth sores were healing and I had reason to hope that I might be on the mend. It was clear I was still quite ill, but I seemed to be stable and my doctor gave me his cell phone number assuring me he was always just one call away. Things weren't good, but I naïvely? confidently? proudly? moved forward...that is until I woke up on November 17.

Daylight was just beginning to illumine the room when I awoke. "Famished" is the best word I can think of to describe my condition. Everyone knows what it feels like to be hungry when we've missed our regular eating schedule. I've also known the signals that the body sends during an extended fast. And, there seemed to be a unique hunger that came upon me a few hours after a marathon as my body demanded nutritional replenishment.

But on this morning, I felt none of those feelings. I can't say for sure, but I imagine it to be the feeling that a man who is beginning to starve to death feels. I had a mixture of deep hunger, panic, and weakness. I *had* to have some food, *now!*

Joanna quickly brought me a bowl of chicken noodle soup. I gulped it down greedily. After I finished, I stood from my bedside and immediately sensed that something was drastically wrong. Whatever was happening in my body had gone to new levels or hit new organs. I fell face first on the bed and told Joanna to call 9-1-1.

Looking back, I'm not sure this was the best decision, but I wasn't able to think clearly. In about the same amount of time as it would have taken us to get to the hospital, an ambulance arrived in our driveway, paramedics came to our door, and Joanna brought them upstairs.

"What's the matter with you?!" one of the paramedics demanded.

"Mr. Stumbo, what's wrong with you! Have you had a heart attack?"

"Why did you call us?!"

As I sat clothed and dazed on the side of my bed, four young men stood in my bedroom shouting at me.

*Why are they yelling at me? Why don't they just take me to the hospital?*

I remember looking up at Drew. He stood tall, strong, and handsome...but angry. He stared at the men in disbelief. These men who had come to help his dad weren't doing anything but talking!

Finally one of them asked me, "Can you get down the stairs by yourself?"

They were reluctant to bring the gurney up the stairs and carry me down. I rallied my strength and made my way down the stairs. It would be the last time I was on my own feet for many weeks.

The paramedics got me into the ambulance, and then we sat in our driveway for a full twenty minutes. I'm not sure of all that they were doing...trying to get vital signs, talking on their radio, filling out paper work. What I did know was that I couldn't believe that I wasn't being taken to the hospital yet.

*Great. I'm going to die in an ambulance in my own driveway!*

Finally, we arrived back at Salem Hospital. By this time, I was in and out of consciousness. I distinctly remember a couple friends each kindly rubbing my freezing feet. The nursing staff tried various methods of getting my temperature and eventually gave up; my temperature having fallen so low it failed to register on their instruments.

A doctor stood before me with the results of my blood work in hand and said, "I've never seen someone with sodium levels so low who is still alive!"

*See, I'm beating the odds. I'm a healthy guy.*

I have only the vaguest memories of what happened over the next few days: An ambulance ride, a new hospital room, a very kind nurse offering me an Ensure/ice cream shake—strawberry flavored—things being hooked up to me, my nephew coming to visit me, and lots of conversation happening around me.

The next clear thought I had wouldn't be for days and would be drastically different. My naïve and proud confidence brought me this far, but a new chapter was about to be written.

# DAYS 32 THROUGH 36
## *FROM JOANNA'S PERSPECTIVE*

During the first few days at OHSU, John was tested for one thing after another. It seemed there was an endless stream of doctors, residents, specialists, and nurses in and out of his room. They asked us question after question about where he'd traveled, what animals he'd encountered, and what he'd eaten during these trips. Though tiring, we understood the necessity of the process and tried to answer to the best of our ability.

John seemed completely miserable. He kept wanting to stand up and the nurses insisted that he stay in bed. It was sad to watch him be so uncomfortable and not know how to help him.

We knew that John's life hung in the balance, but it seemed that what the doctors were doing had stabilized his condition.

However, on Wednesday, John's third day in ICU, everything took a dramatic turn. As I was getting ready to go up to OHSU to be with John for the day, I got a frightening call from our doctor telling me to get up there as soon as I could. John was coughing up blood and might not make it. Frantic and devastated, I called a friend who came immediately. An hour later, as we pulled into OHSU, I remember rushing out eager to get to John.

As I got nearer to the ICU door, however, I remember my feet seeming to turn to lead. I was torn between longing to see my husband—

whose precious life hung in the balance—and being frightened beyond words that he might already be gone. My body kept moving forward however, and I soon learned that, although he was unconscious, he had stabilized somewhat. I don't remember much of what the doctor said except that I should probably get the kids home to see their Dad soon.

In a daze I began to make those calls to Anna and her husband, Jeff, in Phoenix, and to Josiah who was attending a songwriter's school in Martha's Vineyard, Massachusetts. Drew, a high school senior, had heard of his dad's turn for the worse, left school, and was now with me at the hospital.

Throughout that morning and early afternoon the doctors tried to pump medicine into John's body, but his cells refused to absorb the nutrients they so desperately needed. By mid-afternoon, the doctor told me that because of this, his organs were now at risk. If this trend continued, John would die.

The doctor, who struck me as a very knowledgeable and compassionate person, said she only knew of one drug that could possibly jump start John's cells into receiving what they needed. But, it was risky. This powerful medication needed to be given over three days and could cause hemorrhaging anywhere in the body, including the brain. She needed my permission before she could proceed.

I left the room at such a loss...the one person I had made every major decision of my adult life with was unconscious and unable to help me now when I needed him most. I felt alone with a huge weight of responsibility on my shoulders.

*God help me. What should I do?*

A verse I had learned years earlier kept coming to mind throughout that traumatic day, "All the days ordained for me were written in your book before one of them came to be" (Psalm 139:16).

This day was a surprise to me, but it wasn't to God. He knew it was coming. He was in control.

Drew took my hands and prayed with me. I was moved by how my teenage son suddenly seemed so responsible and care-giving.

I called Anna and Josiah again, and told them of the decision I needed to make. I assured them that I would make the decision myself—if something went wrong, I didn't want them to feel they had any responsibility for it—but I wanted their input. They were supportive and encouraged me to do what I thought best.

I also called various friends and family and got more prayer support. I talked to the doctor again and asked her if she would administer the drug to her husband if he were in this position. She thought for a moment and said that she would probably take the risk and use the medication.

Convinced that the drug was our only real choice, I told the doctor to go ahead. At the same time, back at the church, an email was sent to the congregation announcing that there would be a prayer meeting for us that night. Within hours, a thousand people gathered to pray for John's life. People would tell us later that they prayed like they had never prayed before. They called out to God with a powerful sense of unity and intensity. The news also travelled around the globe. Across the world, Christians prayed.

While they prayed, John's body responded to the medication. He wouldn't be free from the drug and its after-effects for five days, but at least it was doing what it was supposed to do.

For the next five days, family and friends poured in from across the country. New information was slow in coming, however, and in spite of running test after test, we weren't getting any clear answers as to why John was so sick. Each day we all seemed to be on edge as we waited to see if John would pull out of this horrible, mysterious situation.

Tension was high. Everyone was anxious. Occasionally someone would lighten the mood, finding a reason to laugh in the midst of the heaviness. But mostly we waited and prayed. And then we waited and prayed some more.

During these days and the ones that followed, the shared suffering with other families of the ICU waiting area created a unique bond between those of us who lingered there, a rare melding of strangers. Crossing economic and racial barriers, we were all in the same poised state of waiting. Each family had someone they loved in a strange zone between life and death.

A dozen times a day, I'd walk down the long, quiet corridor to the room where John's motionless body lay. I was continuously aware as I passed room after room that each one held someone on the precipice of death. It was sobering and frightening to be in the waiting room when other families received news that a loved one had died.

Friday, John's birthday came and went. He remained unconscious. We wondered if he would live to see another year.

The hospital team's inability to solve the case wasn't for a lack of trying. When I went to the cafeteria one day a staff member in a white lab coat pulled me aside. He kindly explained that he wanted me to know that it seemed everyone in the hospital knew about John and was in some way involved in trying to solve his unusual case.

Finally, on Sunday morning, John regained consciousness. It was the happiest day we had had for months, and its joy wouldn't be equaled for over a year to come. There was such celebration and relief. We were almost giddy.

# DAYS 32 THROUGH 36

Wherever I was, I would have loved to have stayed there for a really long time.

Sometimes words—especially words that describe emotions—don't communicate effectively because we are too quick to think we know what the other person means by their use of the word. For example, if I were to tell you that the only memory I have of those days was a deep, deep peace, you might smile and say, "That's nice" or even "That's great!" And, I might respond with frustration that you didn't really understand what I was saying. This isn't your fault, of course, because how can any of us truly understand what another person has experienced?

I'm not hoping you'll understand what I experienced, I'm simply hoping that you won't too quickly assume that you do understand and, by doing so, miss the power of what I'm attempting to describe.

I remember the first time it occurred to me that emotions have depths that are unknown to us . . . dimensions beyond what we've experienced. It was a February night. I was sound asleep in our little apartment in York County, Pennsylvania. The phone rang. I stumbled out of bed, picked up the phone and heard words that would pierce my heart, "John, I'm sorry to tell you that your father has been killed in a car accident tonight in Montana. Your mom is seriously injured and is being airlifted to a hospital in Billings."

I hung up the phone, walked into the next room, laid down on the floor and curled into the fetal position as I cried. I was twenty-six at the time. I had experienced measures of grief before. However, as I writhed on the floor, grief was unveiling layers of my heart that I didn't know existed. I knew a person could hurt, I just never knew a person could hurt so deeply.

And so it was, as I lay motionless in the hospital bed in OHSU's intensive care unit, my body precariously hanging between life and death, with tubes and wires protruding from almost a dozen places, as doctors took every precaution they knew to sustain my life and as thousands of people—many with great sadness and concern—interceded on my behalf, the sole memory I have is of a sensational peace.

I'm not just talking about a contented feeling of satisfaction that you might have after a good day of a restful vacation at the sea, I'm talking about something that feels like it just might resemble heaven.

I'm talking about an experience so rich that for a year afterward, I cried every time I spoke of it.

I'm talking about a feeling so moving that I know I was changed just by virtue of having experienced it once.

I'm claiming that there is a peace awaiting us that is richer, fuller, sweeter, deeper, wider, more beautiful and satisfying than I ever thought possible.

I'm trying to describe an emotion so fulfilling that thinking back to it makes me feel lonely—not the loneliness of being alone or isolated, but the loneliness of finally making it home and then not being able to stay.

People have asked me, "Did you see heaven?"

My answer is, "No, but I believe I felt it."

Later I would joke with the Salem Alliance family, "I had my hand on heaven's doorknob, but I had too many of you pulling me back with your prayers. I didn't have a chance of getting into heaven with all of you people praying for me!"

The congregation laughed, and I'm glad they did. I meant for it to be humorous. But inside, I couldn't deny that I felt a sense of disappointment. I had been so close to the finish line, but was sent back for another lap of the race. I was so close to being home, but was kindly told I couldn't stay there yet.

Recently I attended the memorial service of a friend. She was about my age and became sick about the same time I did. We prayed for each other and encouraged each other in our trials. We felt like we were walking the same path. Yet, our outcomes were very different. While God was welcoming her into heaven, I was at her memorial service speaking on her behalf. I felt tremendously honored to do so, but I had the strange emotion of envy.

The same congregation prayed to the same God at the same time for the same thing: healing. One recipient of the prayer was now standing in heaven and the other was standing behind the church podium feeling oddly out of place. On the printed order of service that night, I scribbled a brief summary of my emotions, "Thousands of people have prayed for my healing. God has honored those prayers. I find myself being in the very odd position of being the least happy about it."

It's not that I'm upset that I'm alive. I'm in no way suicidal. I'm determined to live out all the days He grants to me on this planet.

However, I am tainted. I have been spoiled. I've felt something and perhaps been somewhere—or at least approached somewhere—that to experience it is to be changed.

As I said, wherever I was, I would have loved to have stayed there for a really long time. Someday I will.

# DAY 37

My eyes slowly opened and began to focus. Peering over my bed were faces I loved but hadn't seen for months or even years. My first conscious thoughts were,

*She's from Montana, she's from Minnesota, he's from Tennessee... they've come from all over to see me. I must really be sick.*

At that moment, having been unconscious for almost a week, I had absolutely no idea of what had happened to me. Later, it was strange to learn of all that had been going on around me and within me, and not being "there" for it. People had travelled thousands of miles to see me, yet I never saw them. Tests were run, yet I knew none of it. Monitors, machines, a PICC line, and a catheter had been attached to me and I was completely unaware.

As my consciousness returned, I was unaware of my environment or all the medical equipment surrounding me. Instead, the very first picture I saw was a photo frame of faces. Dear faces. Smiling faces. My sight was still blurry around the periphery, making their faces like a portrait—what beautiful and welcoming smiles!

This was a great gift to me. To be welcomed back to consciousness with this kind of support was amazing. They travelled hundreds, even thousands of miles to stand at my bedside. I was unable to say even a word to them, but their presence there is something I will cherish for a lifetime.

They were excited. Their prayers were being answered. I was waking up and appeared to be in my right mind.

But I had questions...questions I had difficulty asking. At the time I was being kept alive by tubes running down my nose and throat—tubes for feeding and tubes for breathing—making speech impossible.

I motioned for something with which to write. The male nurse uttered a strong caution, stating that we shouldn't get our hopes up because patients like me often try to write but it rarely works.

My family handed me a pen and held the paper for me. I had great difficulty holding the pen and tried to write far too fast. This obviously wasn't working. Drew wisely suggested that I try to write just one letter at a time which I did and the family guessed as I went along. This strategy worked, although now that I see the original piece of paper I have no idea how they deciphered it.

"Am I dying?"

This is what I scribbled. This is what I needed to know. This, of course, put my family in a difficult position. Their basic answer was, "Yes you were, but now you're getting better." They tried to be hopeful. In fact, they were hopeful. They were excited. I was alive and appeared to be thinking clearly.

One great difficulty in crisis and grief is that people are often at differing stages with each other. For five days, these people who love me dealt with doctors and barraged heaven for my life. They stood soberly at my bedside, shed tears, and consoled each other. They fought fears that I would die or if I survived that I'd have brain damage. They had been through traumatic emotions and now, with great relief, saw me awake and communicating. I was alive! I appeared to be in my right mind! This was a good day! Certainly there were more challenges to come, but for now there was a significant sense of relief and joy.

Meanwhile, I was aware of none of this. I was just now hearing the news of my near death. This is quite a blow for anybody, especially a guy who has naïvely believed he's nearly invincible.

Everyone around me seemed happy. Thrilled in fact.

*What's going on? I'm dying and everyone's in a good mood!*

Looking back I understand. I was just now dealing with the news that they had most of a week to process. I've seen the same situation countless times in families going through a crisis, churches going through a staff change, and many other scenarios. Rarely does everyone involved receive the news simultaneously. Sometimes days or weeks separate the announcement. The church board often hears the news of the pastor's resignation a month before the congregation does. They've had a month head start on the grief process and have moved on to a different stage by the time everyone else is just beginning to deal with it. Overlooking this "grief gap" often causes unnecessary hurt.

*How did I get here? What happened to me? Did I bring this on myself? What was I doing before I got sick?*

The questions sprinted in circles around my mind. I'm a problem-solver by nature. I like to fix things and answer questions. Now I had a brain full of questions but limited ability to ask them. To make matters worse, no one really had any answers.

The lack of answers wasn't for a lack of trying. In the words of one doctor, as she was reviewing my files, "I think they ran tests on him for every virus I've ever heard of."

They tested me for AIDS, infectious diseases, and things I can't pronounce. I had multiple skin biopsies, countless blood draws, some sort of spinal tap and two muscle biopsies. (I seriously objected to the second muscle biopsy since the first one had been inconclusive, but the medical staff prevailed assuring me that it was essential and well worth it.) These samplings of my body were sent to labs and specialists far and wide.

Nothing was conclusive. It's nice to hear that you don't have certain conditions and have some things checked off the list, but after a while the uncertainty was unsettling. And, since they couldn't figure it out, my mind kept trying:

*Was it something I ate? Was it my long distance running? Was it from being bitten by a snapping turtle when I was fishing in Minnesota—do these doctors even know about snapping turtles in Minnesota? He bit me hard. He drew blood. What did I do when I was in Brazil? A fruit I sampled in Arizona was rotten, but I spit it out, could it have been that? Maybe my electrolytes got messed up from not handling my long distance running appropriately. I sure wish I could talk to someone about this!*

# AN INCREDIBLE REALIZATION

The powerful peace I had felt faded. The great surprise of seeing my family and friends that had gathered gave way to the disappointment that I couldn't communicate effectively with them. My false-sense of confidence about my good health succumbed to the reality of my situation—I was gravely ill. My body, so accustomed to daily activity, now lay motionless and virtually paralyzed in bed.

I had entered the hospital weighing 190 pounds. Now, with my body unable to properly process fluids, the hospital bed scale revealed that I weighed 260. Some seventy pounds of fluid weight bloated me. I was swollen from face to feet. If the weight gain had been muscle mass, I would have been someone serious to contend with. Instead, it was unabsorbed fluid that stretched my skin and further sapped my strength. I felt like a blob.

For a while, I was convinced that my arms were tied to the bed.

*Why did they have to restrain me? I'm not going to try to pull any tubes out or interfere with their work! I'm not dangerous. Why do I have to be tied down?*

Later I would understand that it was simply that my arms were so bloated and my muscles so weak, I was literally unable to lift them. I was immobile. My own weight was greater than my strength.

I couldn't sit up and examine my own body. I'd get glimpses of myself now and then when they'd roll me on my side or handle me for some reason. I did become aware, however, that my skin was suffering as well.

Skin is amazing. Somehow it expanded to contain my bloated body. Yet, it wasn't happy about my condition. Any touch to my skin would leave indents for a time—like a memory foam mattress. At one point the medical staff considered cutting slits in my skin to release some of the fluid build-up. I was relieved that before they had to do this, my skin started oozing on its own. My skin had become paper thin and at its weakest points became a place the fluid could release. Cracks in my elbows were layered with crust. The nurses attached some sort of bags to my muscle biopsy sites to catch the steady flow of drainage. I was leaking a yellowish, pussy fluid.

I was being fed during this period through a feeding tube that ran up my nose and down my throat. It wasn't painful, but it wasn't something I ever adjusted to. It didn't hurt, it was just *wrong*.

Meanwhile, the staff wanted to see if I could eat or drink…something I was very eager to try. They gave me sherbet at first and then ice chips. I failed to be able to swallow either of them successfully. This was disappointing and frustrating for me, but I didn't understand the ramifications of what was happening.

I wanted the pleasure of eating and, more importantly, the relief of being able to drink liquid or at least suck on ice chips. All of this became forbidden. I would have the dreaded "Nothing by Mouth" notice posted in my room for all medical staff and visitors to see. My lungs, already at risk, could not be threatened by the high likelihood of pneumonia if food or liquid went down my windpipe.

Joanna understood the significance more fully than I did. She had read that when the inter-skeletal muscles are attacked, the condition in its most serious form can move from the arms and torso to the lungs and swallowing muscles. When this happens the patient rarely has long to live.

"He's not out of the woods yet," a doctor would tell Joanna repeatedly over these days, as if she wasn't concerned enough already.

I had come through an intense battle, but no one was claiming that the battle was over. The reality of my condition sobered me.

I couldn't speak to anyone, so the primary "conversation" took place in my own head. Over and over I would replay various scenarios. Looking back, none of them made any sense. My mind concocted strange sets of circumstances and progressions, all of which led to my death. And, every time my final thought would be, *And if I die, I'll be with Jesus, and that will be good.*

With that, my mind and heart would be at peace again. It didn't matter what worried set of circumstances my mind imagined, every time I landed on the assurance that death only meant one thing: I would be in heaven.

I can't imagine how horrible it would be to be on your deathbed without faith. To come to the point of knowing that your life on earth is done without having an assurance of what comes next is deplorable and unnecessary.

The message I believed since my youth stood the test for me. I was taught from my earliest days that a God of love had created this world and even though the people He created rejected Him, He did not reject us. In His great mercy, He offered a way of salvation for us through Jesus Christ. The life, death, burial, and resurrection of Christ were not merely historical occurrences, but God's provision for us to be the recipients of new life. Christ came to this earth for my salvation. Christ died for my sin. Christ conquered death to "free those who all their lives were held in slavery by their fear of death" (Hebrews 2:15).

I believed that message as a child. As a young adult, I questioned the truthfulness of it. But, after wrestling through some issues, came to believe with greater certainty that, in Jesus' words, He is "the way and the truth and the life" (John 14:6).

As a pastor, I had preached this message frequently. It's one thing to preach it from a pulpit; it's another thing to believe it on your deathbed. Now, with my health in a tenuous condition, this faith I had claimed and proclaimed was tested. I'm happy to testify that it held solid.

The condition of my body was failing, but the condition of my soul couldn't have been better. I didn't know what to expect from life, but I was excited about what awaited me in death.

Please accept my testimony: To be on your deathbed and for death to be the least of your worries is a great place to be.

The New Testament author almost seems to mock as he asks, "Where, O death, is your victory? Where, O death, is your sting?" (1 Corinthians 15:55).

The issue of death had been settled. Living, on the other hand, had some complications.

# OH THE PLACES THE MIND CAN GO

Unconsciousness had been a gift. It was a blessing to have no aware-ness of my condition. But now I was quite aware of my situation. My mind worked relentlessly trying to process what was happening.

I was aware of constant movement around me. During this phase at least one nurse was assigned to me full-time: checking monitors, re-filling the bag containing formula, grinding medicines that other patients could have simply swallowed, responding to yet another beep or signal from one of the dozen or so machines to which I was attached, checking IVs, emptying my catheter, dealing with another eruption from my skin, bathing me, and taking care of things I'll never know about. Other nurses regularly came to assist. I had enough needs to keep them all busy.

I remember thinking about how strange it felt to have people dedi-cating their time—making it their life occupation—to take care of me, another human. My survival was dependent upon others. Their calling, their life-effort, was to give me another chance at life. I felt uncomfort-able being on the receiving end, but I was grateful for it.

I could do literally nothing to take care of myself. There was no bodily function that I could do on my own. If my nose itched, I needed someone else to scratch it. If my teeth were going to be brushed, it would only be by someone else's kindness. You get the idea.

All I could do was think—and that, too, was becoming more difficult as the days wore on. Days and nights mixed together. The distinction between sleep and consciousness blurred.

There was never a time when I didn't recognize the people around me. I always knew my family and friends. Names came easily to mind. I quickly began to identify the members of the medical team assigned to me. I took a deep liking to some of them and had negative opinions of others. I knew I was coherent, but I felt a darkness slipping in.

Prayer was even more difficult. I really didn't even know where to start. Though I had taught others about prayer, I couldn't pray myself. Family and friends would have to do the praying for me for a season.

I was at a place that felt so foreign—on a deathbed in an ICU ward—and I didn't know how to respond. It was a disorientation the likes of which I had never experienced.

I was normally the healthy one; now I was dying. I was normally the one visiting people in these kinds of rooms; now I was the one being visited. I was the one who cared for other people; now I was the one receiving care. I was accustomed to being in charge; now I was completely dependent.

I started to become aware that my mind was in a battle of its own.

*Are there really tap dancers on the wall?* I was seeing something—or at least thought I was—and my mind tried to process it.

*No, of course not. There can't be. That's not logical. You're seeing things. They are kind of cool, though. A guy doesn't get to see tap dancers on the wall every day.*

*Where's my family? It must be night. Yes, it's dark. I wonder if I had my birthday yet. Was I unconscious for my birthday? What a place to spend your birthday. It must almost be Thanksgiving. It doesn't look like I'll be eating any turkey this year. What is that nurse doing now? Is she pouring medicine down my back? What is she doing back there?*

My life was lived inside my head and I had growing reason to be concerned about what was going on inside it. A fear started to arise within me: I was losing my mind. I knew that some of my thoughts were coherent. I sensed that others were not. I began to lose my bearings as to which ones were normal and which ones weren't. Reality and delusion intermingled.

For example, I knew that my daughter Anna had come to see me in the hospital. I knew that she ate healthy food. I knew there was a Trader Joe's Grocery Store not too many miles from the hospital and they sold healthy food. I knew that I was sick—but evidently wasn't thinking about the fact that I couldn't swallow—and healthy food would help me get better. I knew that I couldn't walk and that the hospital people probably wouldn't let me go anyway. But, *if Anna could just get a wheelbarrow and sneak me out of here, she could wheel me to Trader Joe's. We could get some real food and I could get better. Anna's sweet. She'd do that for me.*

Drugs. I had never taken any. In ninth grade when our family moved to Billings, Montana, some guys in my school made a strong effort at making me their newest customer. They made great claims about the substances they were shooting, snorting, and inhaling. Frankly, I was susceptible. I was having a hard time connecting with any positive friendships and these guys were consistent at reaching out to me. They would have been happy to include me in their group. I can only credit God's kindness—and my mother's prayers—for keeping me from getting involved with them.

The medical staff gave me no warning, but at some point, they began giving me very high doses of a medication. I was told later it was Prednisone. Whatever it was, it affected my thinking. In their defense, not everyone reacts to these drugs in the same way, and the medical staff believed the high doses were necessary for my survival. What I know for sure is that for five days my mind took me to places from the worlds of fantasy, science fiction, horror, spiritual warfare, comedy, and insanity.

At first I would question what I thought or saw or thought I saw. My concern for my own sanity had reason to grow.

The ICU rooms have curtains that the staff close when they want the patient to have a measure of privacy. These curtains have seams at the bottom. Who knows how many countless hours I stared at those curtains in various stages of being opened or closed. There was so little to look at in those rooms.

On at least one night, I was attacked by black fish that swam in the curtain seams. It really wasn't a concern if only one of them bit you. They were small and didn't do much damage. But, if two of them bit you simultaneously, you died. I wasn't afraid to die; I just didn't think I wanted to die by fish bite.

They had a weakness, however. If you grabbed them in the curtain seams, and gave them a good squeeze, they popped. I wanted my son, Drew, to come and visit me because I knew he'd be a good fish popper.

Later, I would look at those curtains and think, *Wait a minute. There couldn't be any fish in there! What's happening to me?*

*I don't want to go crazy. I've got to hang on. God, please don't let me lose my mind.*

At this time, I was communicating by means of an alphabet tablet. I had been given an electronic device commonly used by children—something like "my baby's first keyboard"—but sadly, my hands were too weak to use it. My mind sent signals that my body could no longer obey.

My family showed incredible patience as they tried to decipher what I wanted to say. The process of using the alphabet tablet was dreadfully slow and laborious. My wife or son would hold the board and point to a row of letters. I was too weak to point. I'd blink or nod when they came to the row of letters that contained the letter I wanted. Then we'd have to agree on the specific letter from the row. My family became amazingly adept at guessing what letter would naturally come next and what word I was spelling after only two or three letters. Every time they would guess a word I had only half spelled, I felt a sense of relief. Who knew that communication could be so laborious and painful?

One day I was vexed. I had to pass a message on to someone immediately. This was urgent! My family saw the anxiety on my face and found the alphabet board. Together, we began the spelling process.

"Is it this first line?"

I shook my head.

"Second?"

No again.

"This line?"

Uh-uh.

"This one?"

Uh-uh.

"So, it's this line."

I nodded.

"Okay, does it start with S?"

I shook my head.

"T?"

I nodded eagerly. *Great, we've got the first letter.*

Through this tedious procedure they kindly continued until we agreed on two more letters: *E-L.*

"Tell? Is the word 'tell'?"

I nodded a relieved yes.

On we plodded: *R-O-N*

"Okay, Ron."

*N-O-T*

*G-O*

*C-L-A-*

"Class?"

*P-O-R-T*

"Ron's not supposed to go to class in Portland?"

I gave my intense agreement and wanted to keep spelling.

*K-I-L-L*

"Ron's going to be killed if he goes to class?"

*Yes, they're getting it. They've got to get this! Ron's life is on the line and if he dies, others will as well. Did they believe me or am I getting that "We're going along with it but just to humor you" look?*

"Who is 'Ron'?"

*I don't think they even know Ron Peters, but they could call the church office and the church staff could get a hold of him.*

*P-E-T-E*

"Oh, Ron Peterson. Okay, we'll go make a call..." the family agreed, and it was clear that our conversation was over.

*No! Ron Peterson is an old friend of ours from college. Ron Peters is from our church choir. It's his life that is in danger.*

I was left alone in my room as they went to make their "call." I knew they hadn't believed me.

*How could they not believe me? This is serious!*

I knew—I had watched it so clearly—this was huge!

*Aliens have invaded our region. They look like normal people but they're not. They have the power to kill a person just by touching them... usually on the chest by the heart. But their weakness is that they are limited in their location. They watch our patterns and behaviors and position themselves at the exact locations that we pass each day. They will be waiting for him at class. But, if he doesn't go, he'll be safe.*

What I couldn't tell Joanna, but made my passion all the more intense, was that she was on the alien hit-list as well. If they got Ron, they'd get the next person. Number three on the list was a nurse I had come to appreciate and Joanna was number four. If we stopped one, we would stop them all.

I lay in my bed strategizing what to do next. People's lives were in my hands, but I didn't know what to do to save them.

Now when I talk about these experiences I explain, "Do you know the difference between a nightmare and a hallucination? When you wake up from a nightmare, you breathe a big sigh of relief and say, 'Wow, I'm glad that was just a dream.' When you wake up from a hallucination you say, 'We've got to do something about this!'"

I know I've forgotten some of the hallucinations, but others are permanently etched on my mind.

For example, I "saw" my breath make fabulous and intricate patterns of the most exquisite material—heavenly fiber-optic swirls of gasses that solidified when you touched them. A miniature and delicate universe was being created in front of me. I watched the shapes with a holy delight.

The Eastern European nations' attempt to take over America by way of nurses who were human in their upper body, but had legs made of Styrofoam was a complex and sometimes frightening plot. I had been implicated in this plot because my own name had been picked up in an illegal passport manufacturing scheme where multiple names were invented based on the letters found in my own name. I assumed that they had stolen the name band that I had on my wrist at some point of this hospital stay.

I did envy the nurses' Styrofoam legs, however. They were so efficient and needed no nourishment. I figured they'd make great marathon runners.

A massive natural disaster had wiped out Africa. I was given a leadership position to assist in the rebuilding of the continent. The elephants, rhinos, and other wildlife had grown to monstrous sizes and were stampeding across the landscape. An epic battle was forming.

Any memory of my past or stimulus around me could be turned into a fascinating adventure. The faces of the leaders of my denomination appear on the game my children once played—Guess Who. The scene changes and I'm buried under a pile of books and magazines and no one knows I am there. I discover I am in the basement of a couple who are harboring refugees of some crisis. Now I'm made to sit on a countertop in a business run by people who are always rushing back and forth but never give me a job to do. I'm just to sit and watch, watch, watch. I don't like being here. I wonder what their business is and what country I'm in.

One story melds into another. To this day I don't know if some of them only lasted for seconds or if they carried on, as they seemed to, for hours and hours. I do know that I spoke of some of them and they continued through "consciousness" and sleep.

A new scenario is before me. I have access to an amazing machine of sorts. If I can operate it correctly or get the calculations accurate, I can reverse human history to sometime in the 1940s and reverse all sin and evil that has taken place on the planet since them. It's working. Evil like waves begins to recede. It pulls back like a great unholy tide. Josiah prays. Great victory and celebration is coming to earth. I want to weep with joy.

Oh, no, now I've stumbled upon a street fair and inadvertently found myself as one of the characters in a street play. It is an existential type of play like something from Sartre that I must have read in high school. The main actors, a male and female nurse, roll me—the patient—back and forth, changing my diaper again and again, rubbing something like sandpaper on my backside. I'm stuck in this drama. It has no plot and no ending. The nurses talk back and forth, they fall in love, they marry and have a child—a lifetime passes and the whole time they roll me back and forth, doing their unending job. I'm trapped on the bed. I'm stuck in the play. It has no meaning. It has no end. The actors are insane. I'm the only one in my right mind, but I'm trapped on this bed, trapped in this story.

I could go on, but don't care to. Other hallucinations were grotesque or bizarre to the degree that I choose not to revisit or record them.

After five days of these experiences, Joanna made a passing reference about my hallucinations to the medical staff. They expressed surprise. They weren't aware that I was struggling in this manner.

They said, "Oh, we can give him something for that."

Another drug was introduced to my system, and within twenty four hours the wild ride was over and my mind gradually returned to normal. However, whatever was attacking my body was still on a wild ride of its own.

# KNOCKING AGAIN ON DEATH'S DOOR

November came to a close as did the visits of the many people who had traveled across the country to see me. Their presence had encouraged me and provided support for Joanna and our kids, but lives had to be lived and flights had to be caught. I had dodged death and they returned home with mixed emotions. I was alive but still a cause for countless prayers.

As the days of December wore on, Joanna, who had been at my side day and night, became concerned that my strength was not improving. In fact, she noticed signs of decline that disturbed her. As two doctors were making their rounds one day, she asked, "How much weaker can he get? When will this turn around?"

They both just stood shaking their heads and admitted that they didn't really know.

The events of these weeks blur together. Joanna and I don't remember the sequence of these events. We just know they happened.

I'm told that I have pneumonia. I'm aware that they are doing a procedure to withdraw fluid from my lungs. I can't watch them because they are doing whatever they are doing to enter my lungs through my back. I hear them say something that piques my curiosity. I ask if I can see the results of their work. I'm stunned to see in their hands a clear container holding at least a liter of ugly fluid that moments ago had been inside of me.

—❧—

The lift team is turning me over as they do every few hours throughout the night. I hate these times. I know they are necessary to prevent me from getting bed sores, but I feel like a slab of raw meat. They grab my unresponsive body, place it in a different position and readjust the pillows supporting me.

Suddenly I'm unable to breathe. Someone notices. Almost immediately, it seems, three doctors and three extra nurses are at my side. They look at the monitors. They look at me. They look at each other. A rapid discussion erupts.

I hear commotion. I don't understand what is happening. The urgency in their voices increases as they deliberate the best course of action. Joanna sees the confusion on their faces and the panic in mine. Suffocation is a terrifying feeling. Someone takes charge. A decision is made. I can breathe again. I dread the next time the lift team must come.

———◦∞∞◦———

I am forbidden to have my hospital bed reclined completely. My head must always be elevated at least thirty degrees. After weeks, I weary of this position. I finally drift off to sleep. An alarm sounds. I'm awakened. I so badly just want to go back to sleep again. Suddenly someone is at my side rapidly explaining that my oxygen has slipped to a dangerously low point and the breathing apparatus I dread reappears. My mouth is opened. The tube is inserted into my throat again. I think they call it being "intubated." I hate this. They say I could have died. I just want to sleep.

———◦∞∞◦———

I have to sign a document granting the medical staff permission to perform a tracheotomy. My breathing has reached a degree of weakness that more extreme measures must be taken. I barely know what this means. I have memories of an old man I once saw at a nursing home—the victim of throat cancer after a lifetime of smoking—whose voice was unnatural, mechanical. They place a pen in my hand. I cannot write anything legible, but it will suffice for their authorization. I can't believe that it has come to this.

———◦∞∞◦———

"He's not thinking clearly here! Mrs. Stumbo, you need to give me permission to do this!"

My oxygen has again slipped to a dangerous level. Respiratory therapists have again rushed to my side.

*Who are these people and where do they come from? Why are they always interrupting my sleep!*

They want to change something regarding my tracheotomy and need my permission. I'm frustrated. I launch into a raspy explanation of why I think this is entirely unnecessary.

This does not settle well with the therapist who insists that even as we speak, I am in danger. He insists that not only is this essential, it is urgent. He claims that I am running out of oxygen.

I feel like I have plenty of oxygen at the moment and don't understand his impatience. Really, I don't understand anything he is saying. I believe I'm fine and want to be left alone. I refuse to give him permission for whatever it is that he wants to do.

It's at this point that he turns to Joanna with his demand. I see the distress on her face. I've put her in a horrible position. She's caught in a fight between the husband she loves and a medical staff she has come to trust.

*Why am I doing this to her?*

My spirit suddenly softens. My stubbornness subsides.

"Go ahead," I whisper.

Within seconds the procedure is done. The staff seems to sulk away. My wife thanks me with a look of deep gratitude.

---

"I hope that's not for Drew's dad," two doctors say to each other as they race down the hall in response to Code Blue. They have been touched by the sweetness that the tall teenager—part tender boy, part full-grown man—has shown to his father. To their dismay the code is for me.

They rush in. Decisions are made. Orders are given. Drew's dad's life is spared again.

---

"Mrs. Joanna Stumbo. Mrs. Joanna Stumbo. Please return to ICU."

Joanna's heart sinks as she rushes out of the cafeteria, her lunch interrupted by the voice over the loudspeaker. With heart and mind racing, she reaches the nurses' station to be told, "We need your signature."

With a deep sigh of relief, she signs the form.

---

Joanna and Drew have put in another long day together at the hospital. I've had a fairly good day and seem stable. They get home to Salem a little before midnight. Joanna sets her phone on the counter and catches a quick shower. When she gets out, a message is waiting on her phone. She returns the call. It is promptly transferred to the young female doctor whom the family has come to deeply respect and appreciate.

With a compassionate tenderness in her voice, the doctor gently breaks the news,

"John's not responding. We've had to re-intubate him. You need to come immediately."

Within minutes, mother and son are back in the Saturn and back down the same long road they have just travelled. Drew, a cautious driver for a male his age, quietly listens to melancholy sounds of *Coldplay* as he makes his way back to the interstate. Joanna stares out the passenger window desperately trying not to cry. For Drew's sake, she attempts to keep her composure. She has cried many tears alone, but hasn't yet broken down in front of the kids—it's her mother's heart, ever protecting her children.

Quietly, she considers what seems to be the inevitable: *John's cheated death too many times. He can't possibly do it again. This has to be it. He's gone.*

The miles wear on. The weariness of this battle, already weeks old, weighs upon her. Finally, the waves of emotion wash over her.

Sobs pour out—gasping sobs. Staring out into the emptiness of the night, she fears that she has become a widow. It becomes one of the longest drives she has ever endured.

Shortly after 1:00 am, mom and son rush back into the ICU ward with which they are now all too familiar. The gentle doctor is seated on the side of my bed, my hand in hers.

Cautiously, but with hope in her voice, she explains that I have started to respond again. I have squeezed her fingers. Once again I am pulling out of it.

For the next hours, I lay completely motionless, showing no signs of consciousness. Instead of getting a night of sleep in her own bed, Joanna spends another night at my bedside, fearing that I've experienced brain damage, longing for me to respond to her presence in some way, but relieved that death had passed me by again.

Months would pass before I would hear the full story of what I had put her through that night and others like it. As throughout my entire journey, she would deflect attention away from herself. She was fighting for me. She refused to let the story become about her. She would receive people's sympathy, but then quickly defer back to the man to whom she had said her vows—vows that were being tested.

Her faith was being tested as well. There were two very specific times she felt she was on the edge of despair. The "water" of our crisis seemed to have risen to a level that might drown her. Once, on a rare night when she was alone at home in bed, trying to get a real night of sleep, she felt the despair threatening to overwhelm her. A second time, walking the skywalk between two hospital buildings—feeling alone and discouraged—wondering if we'd ever get out of this crisis or leave these buildings, the waters seemed too deep. Each time she cried out in her spirit, *You promised not to let the waters flood over me. I feel like I'm about to drown.*

Both times, within the hour, God met her and she found herself in a completely different emotional state. Verses she had heard so many times through the years kept coming to mind and became anchors of hope, foundations of faith:

*We are hard pressed on every side, but not crushed; perplexed, but not in despair; persecuted, but not abandoned; struck down, but not destroyed* (2 Corinthians 4:8-9).

*When you pass through the waters, I will be with you; and when you pass through the rivers, they will not sweep over you. When you walk through the fire, you will not be burned* (Isaiah 43:2).

In many other ways and at many other times, Joanna and I would be strengthened directly by God's Word. Often times this came via God's people; but even this was not simple. Wisdom would be needed as to which voices we should listen to.

# GUESTS AND GIFTS

A guy like me doesn't take off his "pastor" hat easily. I've been "Pastor John" since I was twenty. There are probably many reasons why pastors don't always make the best patients, but one of them came as a surprise to me: I felt like I was somehow responsible to host or entertain everyone who came to visit. I was grateful that they came to see me, but felt pressure to keep the conversation going. Even when I had no ability to speak, I still felt responsible for what took place around me.

The one exception was when I sensed that the person had come to see me without expecting anything from me.

For example, one of my sisters and her husband waited until the initial flurry of activity had subsided and then came to visit. When she stood at my bedside, hour after hour for most of a week, I knew I didn't have to talk. She may have come right out and explained it to me. I'm not sure. But what I do know is that I sensed, "John, you don't need to say anything. I'm just here to be with you."

I relaxed. I asked her for help. At my request, the room temperature was set as low as the thermostat would allow: 55 degrees. With only a hospital gown and thin sheet covering me, I still felt like I was burning up. Time after time, my sister cooled my raging face and forehead with a freshly dampened washcloth.

I asked her to sing. Hymns I hadn't heard for years were kindly and quietly sung over my bed. One song I had never heard before became my most frequent request:

*There is a healing stream from the hand of God,*
*Enter in, enter in.*

My mind could not handle any significant visual stimulation. Television was dreadful. Far too many images per minute raced by for me to process. It was wearisome. But gentle music was soothing and no music more so than that of my son. When Josiah would bring his guitar, sit on the floor by my bed with his back against the wall, for a brief moment I could picture that we were back home together as a family. All was well. Dinner had just been enjoyed and Josiah would pull out his guitar, sit down on the carpet, lean against the wall, and play a song. I loved those moments and was grateful when he brought them right into my ICU room.

Others, like my brother-in-law, didn't sing, but had a scripture to share and a prayer to pray. He respectfully brought me his contribution and then slipped out.

My eighty-nine-year-old mother, who had spent months of her life in a bed just like this, kept slipping into my room even when the staff was trying to keep everyone away. My mom, the eighty-nine-year-old sneak! With cane in hand, she would stealthily slip away from the other family members, out the lobby, down the corridor, past all the nurses, doctors, and staff to quietly stand at my bedside. She might touch my arm and no doubt prayed silent prayers, but I don't think a word was spoken. My weak voice and her weak hearing made communication impossible anyway, but it didn't matter. It wasn't why she was there.

Some communication is best done without words.

On a different day, another lady slipped passed the nursing staff as well. Although I had only met her once before, I recognized her immediately. She set a bouquet of flowers on the window ledge, came to my bed and said, "Pastor Stumbo! Do you want to die? Are you trying to die?!"

As a pastor, I have always welcomed into my office anyone who wants to see me. I may not be able or willing to allow them a second appointment, but I'll meet with anyone once. This woman, her husband, and ten-year-old son had come to visit me some weeks before I became ill. They met with me to inform me that I—and my entire congregation— were living in sin because we were not following the Old Testament food regulations.

Her rebuke and challenge took me back to a study of scriptures and I was reassured that Jesus had pronounced all foods clean and that the righteousness that Christ now brings us surpasses that which could be attained through the law. The New Testament church was not based upon the ancient Jewish rituals and regulations. Our Christian faith, while greatly enriched by our Jewish heritage, is not bound by it.

I hadn't heeded her admonition. I had rejected her counsel. I had done so graciously, attempting to explain to her my understanding of the scriptures. Yet, I hadn't backed down and, yes, I still had pepperoni on my pizza.

Now she was standing at my bed. My sudden and unexplained illness made perfect sense to her. She informed me that I had hardened my heart to the Word of God that she had spoken to me. I was living in sin and leading other people down the same path. If I did not repent, I would die. It was as simple as that.

Her son, a tender boy that my heart went out to, watched from the nursing station window.

Little else was said. She placed a card on my chest and had me promise I would read it. I assured her I would. I never saw her again.

*Could she be right? God, is this really what my illness is all about? Have I sinned against you by what I've eaten? Am I wrong? I'm willing to confess any sin of which you convict me. Am I missing something here, God? I'll study the passages all over again when I get well. But God, I can't imagine that this is what my illness is all about. Please, if I'm wrong, let me know. Otherwise, I'm assuming it is okay with you that I ignore her rebuke.*

I would keep the promise I made to myself. I did review the relevant scriptures after I was released from the hospital. But I will admit that the ordeal was unsettling. I wanted to be open—and still do—to anything God would want to say to me. But today, as throughout all of church history, discernment is needed. Not everyone who claims to speak on behalf of God actually does. The scriptures are full of warnings about false prophets. Yet, I don't want to be guilty of disregarding someone God has sent to me just because they have a message I don't want to hear or a methodology I don't like.

A few weeks later, another visitor would give me another opportunity to seek discernment.

We had a constant stream of visitors for weeks. Many of them weren't able to come to my room, but Joanna welcomed them in the lobby. They brought with them cards, prayers, food, and encouragement.

However, by mid-December a historic snow and ice storm blanketed the entire area. For days freezing rain pummeled us. Then came the snow. Then more freezing rain. Inches of dangerous ice covered the roads. It became impossible for crews and plows to keep up. For over a week travel was almost impossible. The storm finally subsided, but it left an entire region paralyzed.

During this time I didn't see hardly anyone except Joanna, the boys, and the hospital staff. I pitied the staff who had to work around the clock, unable to go home as their replacements couldn't make it in to work. I pitied Joanna who had to spend four days in the same set of clothes and wash her hair in the bathroom sink. I never heard her utter a complaint.

The only outside visitor we had for a stretch of those stormy days was a man we had never met. I'm embarrassed to admit that Joanna and I were cold toward him at first.

He appeared to be about my age, maybe a little younger. He had a kind face, gentle demeanor, and what I call "a Pacific Northwest earthiness" about him. He spoke in low tones.

He introduced himself apologetically, admitting that the only way that he had been allowed into my room was by telling the hospital staff that he was a family member.

"But, I am your brother in Christ," he defended.

Here he stood. Unknown. Uninvited. I wasn't overly receptive. Discouragement had settled in to my spirit by this time. He had certainly arrived at a low point.

*We're not getting off to a very good start. Who is this guy anyway?*

He seemed nervous. He explained that he had heard about our crisis and felt God telling him that he was supposed to come and pray for me. Joanna, feeling uncomfortable with this stranger in the room, asked him a few questions about himself. She was simply trying to figure out who this visitor was. It seemed that what he really wanted to do was get right to prayer.

*Whoever he is, he's braved horrible roads to be here. I'd be happy to have him pray. What can it hurt?*

He started his prayer in English, but didn't stay there very long. I had heard people use a prayer language or speak in tongues many times, but I had never heard anything like this.

He prayed one word at a time. Carefully. He didn't seem to be speaking in sentences, but in single words—each one specifically chosen—or was he listening for them? The words were fascinating to hear. They struck me as an odd guttural combination of sounds which seemed to me to have a high ratio of consonants to vowels. They were thick. Sturdy. Robust.

His pauses were so long that at one point Joanna started talking, assuming his prayer was over. He continued on. I wondered, *God, what kind of prayer is this? Is this of you? What do I do with this?*

It is my conviction that the Holy Spirit is still gracing Christ-followers with the same gifts He did in the New Testament times. I've witnessed their effective use. I find no scriptural basis for expecting Him to do any less in the twenty first century than He did in the first century.

I've sought to speak in tongues myself at times. A godly Pentecostal pastor friend of mine had prayed over me years earlier that I would receive the gift. I eagerly opened my heart and mouth to whatever God chose to give me. I would not pretend. I would not attempt to make something up on my own. I would pray and wait and accept God's decision on the matter. I know I disappointed my pastor/brother, but I left our encounter as mono-lingual as I came. Yet, I had a peace. The Spirit gifts us as He chooses (1 Corinthians 12:11). Tongues is a beautiful gift. It just wasn't mine to have.

I'm open to the use of spiritual gifts. I'm also aware that there can be misuses. I had worshipped in a few churches through the years where I questioned the validity of their practices. I prayed,

"God, forgive me if I'm wrong. I'm just trying to wade my way through truth and error, real and counterfeit. If it's of you, I want to be part of it. If it's not, I don't want to be fooled."

And so, once again being stretched by a new experience, as I looked up into this stranger's face from my hospital bed, I silently prayed, *God, is this of you? Are you in this? What he is doing is counter to all of my experience and outside of my comfort zone, but is he your servant, doing your will? Did you bring him here to stand at my bedside to do what he's doing?*

As he finished his prayer, he gently spoke the words, "Today, your healing has begun."

I delight that thousands of people were praying for me—that heaven was being bombarded with my name. I really don't know that God used this man's prayer any more than he used anyone else's. Nor do I know if anything happened in my body at that moment.

What I do know is that something happened in my heart: Faith was born.

His words seemed to be more than sounds landing on my ears. They seemed to take on substance, form together, and become a single speck landing on my heart. A seed of faith had been sown.

I would suffer more setbacks. I would shake the handle on heaven's door another time or two. My recovery would be long and trying...but somewhere in the soil of the soul something had been planted.

He left as silently as he came. I never saw him again. The seed of faith he left behind would seem to lie dormant for weeks. Circumstantially, everything looked the same when he walked out the door as when he walked in. I was still in the same body, connected to the same machines, fighting the same issues, but somehow I had hope that a corner had been turned.

I wasn't trying to make myself believe it. I wasn't trying to convince myself of it. I saw no evidence of it. But a word had been spoken, and the word seemed to have substance.

Joanna, too, would look back at that moment and wonder if the question she had asked the doctors—"when will this turn around?"—had just been answered.

Perhaps the storm had subsided. Perhaps the worst of its rampage was over. We might have to live with the "icy" results for a while, but perhaps the day of healing had begun.

# IS HE OKAY?

More than a week had passed since my hallucinations subsided. I now had enough tubes out of my throat that I could talk. And, what I had to say seemed to make sense to others. Family and friends breathed sighs of relief that I hadn't lost my mind, and it seemed that I was processing information appropriately.

Joanna, however, was still a bit concerned. Granted, I had given her reason to be. For example, there was the night when I was so tremendously uncomfortable that I began to complain about how they had me propped up in bed. The nurses were taking appropriate measures so that I would not develop bed sores, but I had been positioned in an unnatural angle and didn't like it.

"They've got pillars under me!" I groaned.

Joanna looked concerned, "They've got what?"

"Pillars!" I demanded.

She left the room to find someone from the medical staff. I knew immediately what she was up to and I was mad.

A doctor came in and with concern asked the routine questions, "Where are you right now?"

"OHSU."

"What city are you in?"

"Portland."

"What year is it now?"

"2008."

"Who is the President of the United States?"

*Ah, trick question,* I thought.

"Bush is still president, but Obama has been elected."

Satisfied that I was in my right mind, the doctor left and I scolded Joanna, "See, I'm not losing it!"

"You said you had pillars under you and you've said other things that seemed weird, so I just had to make sure you weren't hallucinating again."

I wasn't satisfied with her answer at the time, but looking back later, I realize how fragile my mind still was during those weeks. I thought I understood far more than I really did…but then again, maybe there was nothing new about that. I've always had an abnormally high level of confidence in what I think I know; but at this stage of my recovery, my confidence wasn't serving me well.

"Did you guys know they can put a sports car on that thing?" I commented to my sons one day.

"No. Really?" they both said with surprise.

I had been painfully propped up in a chair for a half-hour a day to begin to rebuild my strength and give me a change of scenery. My fifth floor view allowed me to look out over the gray skies and gray snow left behind by a blizzard the week before. I knew that the view was meant to inspire, but for me it depressed. The gray world matched my gray spirit.

The only thing that gave the scene variety was the occasional arrival of the OHSU tram. I had never ridden it and didn't know where it released its passengers, but I understood its function. Somehow though, probably as I dozed off in my chair, I "saw" a fabulous sports car—Formula One style—attached to the side. Wheels up, affixed as with a massive magnet, the car rode all the way to the top. I doubted that my boys had seen it, and I thought they'd be interested.

They're accustomed to believing their father—good sons that they are—and took my word for it…at least until they walked away.

"Hey, wait! They can't put a sports car on that thing. There's no way!" They concluded the obvious before they got down the hallway.

I realized the same thing myself when, a few days later, they gave me my first wheelchair ride and let me sit in the lobby area where the tram passengers disembark. It's a strange feeling to realize that what you believed you knew to be true was actually the creation of your own imagination. I felt embarrassed like a child who had said something silly in the presence of adults, and promised myself I'd be more careful in the future with what I said to others.

Meanwhile, the family had reason to keep an extra eye on me. Was I really coherent or not?

It was around this time that I was moved to a different ICU room. The nursing staff rolled me in on my bed with my ever-faithful wife accompanying them. The staff left the two of us alone.

I saw it first.

Above me was a strange configuration. Suspended from the ceiling, right over my head, was a fairly large multi-armed steel contraption. I assumed it was for a patient in traction.

Joanna saw it as well and tried to distract my attention from it. In my mental state, she had reason to fear what I could imagine it to be. If I had made the nursing staff out to be Eastern European spies and could hang sports cars from trams, what would I make of this monstrosity?

At that moment Drew walked in, looked up and said, "Whoa! What is that?"

I saw Joanna give him that quick, motherly "be quiet" look, but it was too late. Game on. I saw my chance, "It's a mind-altering machine," I said.

Drew just stared at me while Joanna's heart sank and she let out a groan. I burst into one of the few laughs I had enjoyed in weeks.

"Just messing with your heads," I admitted. "I think it's for traction."

Later she would laugh—months later—but for now it was enough to know that her husband was back in sound enough mind to make a joke.

Sadly, in the days to come, the opportunities to laugh were hard to find.

# BACK TO SALEM

"We'll just have to call it the Stumbo Syndrome."

As the OHSU doctor gave me my release, she acknowledged the mystery of my condition, "You've stumped us all."

I couldn't help but smile to myself as she said those words. After running over a hundred tests on my body, one of the finest medical teams in the region was still puzzled. I found it fascinating. Since then, however, I have had hundreds of people express surprise and disappointment to me, "You mean they never figured out what it was?"

Some people have seemed almost appalled that the doctors hadn't solved the case.

We expect so much out of the medical community...too much. They don't always have answers and we certainly don't want them to pretend they know more than they do. I view the lack of a definite diagnosis as simply a part of what God was doing. I take it as a sign that more was going on than meets the eye. I take genuine comfort in my belief that God knows exactly what is going on at all times, and when He chooses to keep us in the dark on a matter, He does so with purpose. The lack of a clear diagnosis was also a part of His plan.

The staff, it seems, had run out of tests to run and I was no longer in critical condition, so they honored our wishes to transfer me back to Salem. I was still very sick but there was nothing OHSU could do for me that a smaller hospital couldn't handle and I wanted to be closer to home. Travel would be easier for my family. I would find comfort, I assumed, from more familiar surroundings.

The temperature was still below freezing as the ambulance crew wheeled me out the exit. It had been so long since I had smelled something so wonderful. Air. Fresh air. Frigid, damp, Pacific Northwest fresh air. I asked if I could stay there outside the hospital door as long as possible. The attendant kindly agreed as the driver left us to retrieve the ambulance. I breathed as deeply as my damaged lungs would allow. My skin grew cold but I didn't care. It was the closest I had felt to being alive for some time.

The last two months of decline, pain, tubes, needles, tests, biopsies, hallucinations, and being confined to a hospital bed were perhaps coming to a close. Maybe there was reason to hope.

All too soon my thoughts were interrupted as I was wheeled into the stark and sterile confines of the ambulance and my momentary pleasure was over.

The ambulance ride was one to remember. It had taken the hospital staff the better part of a week to find someone willing to transport me. The storm had left thick layers of ice across wide swaths of the Pacific Northwest and Interstate 5 between Portland and Salem was still an ice rink. We bounced and jerked as we slowly made our way over the ruts and ridges created by ice. The attendant's head nearly hit the ceiling on more than one bounce. The driver cursed as another vehicle swerved out of control in front of him. My discomfort and irritation increased by the mile. No one was happy.

Having driven the same stretch of road countless times, I tried to imagine where we were. I could see nothing out the windows from my position, flat on my back, strapped to the bed.

"Are we to Woodburn?" I asked hopefully, referring to the last town before we reached Salem.

"We're only to Wilsonville," came the discouraged reply.

I had missed my guess by fifteen miles.

Finally, two hours later, we arrived in Salem. It was Christmas Eve. I insisted that my family go to church. I'm not sure why. Maybe it was because this had become my favorite service of the year to lead as a pastor.

I think I wanted life to get back to normal. I was trapped in this body, connected still to a half-dozen pieces of equipment, bed-ridden and feeling horrendous, but maybe if others could just go do what I longed to do, perhaps I would find some solace.

It didn't work very well. Discouragement was setting in. I was now conscious enough to be fully aware of my situation. I discovered that something rivaled the hallucinations in its difficulty: reality. Awareness brought with it great challenges.

My family did their best to bring Christmas to my room. Our married children, Jeff and Anna, had come in from Phoenix. Our boys were both home as well. The six of us did our best to be cheerful...but I couldn't get past the heaviness that I felt hanging over me. I didn't want to celebrate Christmas this way. I didn't want to be here. I didn't want to be sick.

My fingers weren't strong enough to remove the wrapping paper. My spirit was not strong enough to truly celebrate. I—who had helped entire congregations rejoice in the coming of the Christ child—couldn't bring myself to enter in. The contrast of Christmas presents and the hospital environment—complete with electrodes attached to my chest, PICC line under my skin, feeding tube in my stomach, spit suction in my mouth, tracheotomy in my throat, etc—was too much for me. I just wanted Christmas to be over. I wanted all of this to be over.

Dr. Byrkit, my local primary care physician, came to the hospital to visit me before leaving for vacation. I was grateful to have a few moments alone with him. He was encouraged by my improvements, but was concerned about something he saw in my chart.

"John, your chart says that you have a DNR—Do Not Resuscitate."

I nodded. I was weary from this battle. "If I have another setback, just let me go."

I don't know how my voice sounded, but my heart was pleading with him.

His puzzled face said as much as his words.

I knew I had disappointed him. What I didn't understand, and he patiently tried to help me understand, was that there were good indicators that the disease activity was subsiding. I had solid medical reason for hope of improvement. I was getting better. He believed I'd be well enough to be on my feet and walking in a few months. This was no time to give up hope.

However, Dr. Byrkit, a follower of Christ, didn't stop there. He went on to tell me that he believed God wasn't done with me or my ministry. He had more work for me to do and wasn't ready for me to go home. This was no time to give up. He appealed to my Stumbo-hard-working-determination. He wanted me to dig deep and make efforts at my own recovery. God had more for me, but I needed to be a willing participant.

It seemed the pastor was getting a solid sermon from the doctor. He even threw in a "sermon illustration" citing a recent movie and challenged me to "prepare for rain."

I listened with mild irritation. I wasn't angry with him because I knew he had my best interests in mind and was speaking his heart to me. I just knew that I didn't have the same level of confidence that he did in my own recovery.

*I don't think I could do all this again. If I have another setback, I'll end up a vegetable.*

In God's mercy, my instructions were irrelevant as I would not physically slip that low again. Emotionally, however, my battle was just beginning.

I never knew how much being able to talk meant to me until that ability was taken away. I had endured weeks of that speechless condition at OHSU, but by the time I reached Salem, I had been able to speak—weak and raspy though it was—for some time.

However, on more than one occasion after Christmas, my oxygen levels would slip into a dangerous zone, an alarm would go off at someone's desk and staff would come running to once again readjust the tracheotomy. To this day, I still don't understand the system of different valves and processes used. All I know is that I absolutely dreaded when they would once again put me on the more extreme forms that disabled my ability to speak.

"Is there anything you need to say before we replace the valve?" I was asked.

What do you say when you only have a moment to say it? I mumbled a few words I no longer remember, they made the adjustments, and I entered the coffin of silence again. I had been here so many times before—trying to communicate with a reader board or a blink of my eyes. It felt so isolating. So lonely. Suffocating.

Nurses, for the most part, were kind and didn't mind playing the guessing game, "Do you need a blanket? Are you cold?" I was frustrated by the nurses who assumed they knew what I needed and appreciated the ones who actually looked at me, trying to sense what my need might be. Worse were the ones who would say something like, "Do you need a drink?" and then remember, "Oh, you can't have anything, can you."

Most of the nursing staff was fantastic, however. True concern showed on their faces. True care was given to me. True comfort was found in their kindness. Later I would write in a blog entry, *Blessed are the caregivers, for in them we have seen the Christ.*

One night, we were all put to the test. I had just started to slip off to sleep when a nurse came in and asked what I needed. I was able to speak again by this time of my hospital stay.

"I'm fine."

"But, you rang the call button."

"Oh, I'm sorry; I must have bumped it by accident."

A few minutes later, she was back asking again how she could help. I assured her I hadn't called her and didn't need anything.

By the fourth and fifth time this happened, we were all frustrated. I wanted to sleep and kept being bothered by nurses who kept being called into my room only to have me deny that I needed anything.

Then my television turned on by itself. I couldn't handle the stimulus of television and certainly didn't want it on when I was trying to sleep. My hands weren't strong enough to handle a remote control, but I didn't have to wait long for a nurse to help me because my call button had buzzed again. At least this time I had something to ask help for.

By now, the staff realized that something was wrong in my room and that I wasn't just pestering them. Then the TV turned itself on again and started rapidly changing channels. That's when maintenance was called. It was well past midnight, but from somewhere in the building the night shift guy came to problem solve. He tinkered and muttered. It was determined that I would have to change rooms.

I wasn't too happy about this because not only did it mean that my sleep would be delayed longer, but I'd have a different nursing staff. I had just had some character-building and memory-making moments with the other nurses, and now I had to start over again with a new crew.

They located a room, wheeled me down the hall, handed me off to a new staff, and wished me good night. A few minutes later a new nurse came in and asked what I needed.

"I'm fine," I assured her.

"But you pushed the call button," she explained.

Oh, this again. From there my memory of the night is kind of a blur. How many more times the TV went on and call button buzzed, I'm not sure. What I do know is that by about sunrise they determined that my bed was the cause of the problem and they'd have to find me a different one.

I know it is often said that hospitals are tough places if you want to get some sleep. Such was certainly the case for me, especially the night my bed went berserk.

Then came the day when the physical therapy department determined that I was healthy enough to stand up…something I hadn't done for six weeks. Three therapists attended me. I was nervous…afraid…yet excited. They gently guided me to the side of the bed and coached me. My world went into slow motion.

Gradually, ever so gradually, I rose up off the bed. I looked straight ahead at the white board where the nurses and aids write their names and what day it is. It is one of the few things to look at in a hospital room and I had stared at such boards from flat on my back for countless hours. Now I was seeing it from a different angle. Higher and higher I stood. I remember thinking, *I didn't know I was this tall*. They coaxed me to rise a little higher still—stand straight, stand taller. I soon began to feel dizzy. They sat me down gently. The whole ordeal had probably lasted less than thirty seconds.

But for me, it was almost as good as a marathon finish line. My fear that I would be permanently confined to beds and wheelchairs was now gone. It was a breakthrough not only for my body, but for my spirit…both of which were about to get a good workout in what awaited next.

# RECOVERY'S STARTING LINE

It's not what I had expected. My first reaction was disappointment. It felt like just another hospital room and I had already spent two months in hospital rooms.

During my bed-ridden weeks in ICU, I imagined a place where I could begin to get some physical exercise. I knew there had to be a facility where people like me could start the rebuilding process. I pictured a large room, full of exercise equipment and therapists. It would have tiny little dumbbells for guys who were starting over. I imagined that adjacent to the workout area were some dorm style rooms and a cafeteria. When I wasn't eating and sleeping, I'd be working out. I would get better. I would be strong again.

As one-by-one tubes and needles, monitors and machines were removed from me, I began to hear the medical staff talk about this mysterious place called "rehab." I had feared that between the hospital and my home I'd be placed in some type of nursing home facility. I dreaded the thought of ending up in one of those rooms I had visited so often as a pastor. On the other hand, I had never been in a rehab unit, but it sounded hopeful.

Of course, I knew that my body had been decimated and that I'd be unable to do the things I had done just months before. Drew and I would regularly go to the YMCA and challenge each other in how many pull-ups and push-ups we could do. The bench press—the male ego lift—was a great rivalry between us. I was slightly ahead of him on that one—maxing out at 225 pounds. He would blow me away on other lifts. It didn't really matter who was stronger. It wasn't about competition; it was about so much more. We'd laugh, we'd push each other, we'd sweat, and we'd grow stronger together on multiple levels. I loved those days.

But now, as I was released from the hospital and admitted to the local rehabilitation center, it wasn't how I envisioned it. First of all, I never imagined that I would leave the hospital in a condition of being unable to swallow, drink, or eat. The concept that one could begin to resume normal life without food and beverage had never entered my mind. There was a cafeteria, as I had imagined, but I would never participate in what they provided. My "meals" were delivered to my room by way of a few cans of a yellowish-green liquid that were poured into a bag and slowly dripped into my feeding tube. I felt isolated.

Second, I underestimated just how weak I was. I could do almost nothing for myself when I first got to rehab. I needed help getting out of bed, getting dressed, using the bathroom, etc. I hadn't imagined that getting back to normal life would be so incremental. The rehab center did have an exercise room, but the equipment wasn't what I had pictured. I wanted a full workout room like a health club; what they had was a therapy room. Despite my disappointment, what they had was exactly what I needed.

My head had said that by the time I got there, I'd be able to do some of the things I once did. Sure, I knew I'd be weak and have to start small…but I had no idea how small.

The first weight that I lifted was a one pound dumbbell. I didn't know dumbbells were made that small. It looked about the size of a dog biscuit. I was embarrassed, yet I knew the therapist was wise in giving it to me. Starting over would not only be physically painful, it would be humbling as well.

"Range of motion" became an important phrase as the occupational therapist gently started me out each day by working my shoulders. I was unable to raise my arms above my head without her assistance. She was kind and spoke gently as she'd guide my arms through the various motions. It seemed to me that she was the one getting the real workout. Our times together always ended too quickly.

Next came speech and swallow therapy. The veteran therapist tested me for memory loss and did useful speech exercises. But for me, these were secondary to the work I really wanted her to do: I desperately wanted to swallow!

I looked forward to her arrival each day, hoping she would bring with her tiny amounts of food or beverage—7-up, yogurt, or pudding. On the days she did, she would administer these to me with great caution and carefully monitor me as I attempted to swallow. Each day my hope would rise that today would be the day that I would begin to eat again.

My efforts were never successful, and she'd always take the food away much too soon for my liking. I wanted to suck on the flavor, but the risk of aspiration and the resultant pneumonia wasn't worth the momentary pleasure I'd receive…at least according to the therapist.

Next came physical therapy. The therapist was feisty, stubborn, and wonderfully optimistic. I fought her as if she were a sister I had known for a lifetime. I was accustomed to figuring out my own workouts. In time, I came to realize that I was in the hands of a well-trained professional who had an amazing ability to know what I was capable of and what I wasn't. In the meantime, I questioned most everything she said.

She was determined to help me walk again. First she assessed my situation. Just months earlier, I had run marathons but I was now being tested to see if I could walk a couple steps without the aid of a walker. The answer was clearly no.

Twice a day she'd work me. Twice a day I'd need a nap afterward. This road to recovery wasn't going to be easy.

# FRIENDS OF MANY KINDS

Late in the afternoon and in the early evening, guests would often stop by the rehab center to visit. I was grateful to hear news of what was happening outside of my little world and receive their encouragement.

Visits felt so much more natural now that I wasn't in a bed looking up at everyone standing around me. Even though I was in a wheelchair, I could at least look them in the eye and just be another person in the circle of peers. I've never had a problem with hundreds of eyes looking at me when I'm on a platform preaching, but after a while I hated being the focus of attention on the hospital bed. I was more relaxed now that I could visit from a chair.

Even better than the conversation, though, was the wheelchair ride that my friend, Steve, took me on one night.

"Want to go fast?" he asked with a mischievous look in his eye.

With our wives engaged in conversation and the nurses nowhere to be seen, Steve gave me a NASCAR tour of the hallways. I don't think I exaggerate when I say that we took some of the corners on two wheels. It felt so good to feel wind in my face again. My only regret was that the rehab halls were so short.

I hated being in a wheelchair, but if I had to be there, we might as well take it for a ride.

Weekend nights were quieter. On these nights, Joanna and I would often find ourselves in a conference room at the end of the hall where an old piano rested in the corner. I don't know why it was there or if anyone ever used it, but on quite a few nights I'd have Joanna close the door behind us, wheel me up to the keys, and with one hand I'd pick out the melody of some old songs—songs that I found waiting for me deep down in the mine shaft of suffering.

*Day by Day* was one of them. The song offered strength to me with its simple melody and lyrics,

"Day by day and with each passing moment,
Strength I find to meet my trials here."

Like an old friend coming to sit by me for a few minutes, the song brought comfort and breathed hope to my weary soul. Even though I couldn't remember all the words, the melody alone whispered its message to me. When my sister, Dori, came to visit me days later, I asked her to play and sing the song in full. Sweet moments. Sweet memories.

A second song I attempted on my own and later requested that my sister sing was *He Giveth More Grace*. Again, I couldn't remember all the lyrics on my own, but the melody brought healing in and of itself; and the lyrics I could recall were like sustenance for the soul.

"When we have exhausted our store of endurance...
Our Father's full giving is only begun."

There in my wheelchair, accompanied by an IV pole—my throat still bandaged to cover the opening from the tracheotomy, my voice barely audible, and my spirit bearing the weight of my mounting losses—Joanna and I sat in the solemn quietness of a rehab unit and let the tears flow with the melody. With our "store of endurance" completely exhausted, we turned to the only place we knew to go—His grace...His grace delivered to us in the package of an old song.

New songs are good. New songs give new expressions of the faith. New songs give outlets to all the creative song writers who reflect the ever-creative Composer Himself. New songs have their place. For good reason—for manifold reasons—the scriptures often declare, "Sing to the Lord a new song."

However, there are times when a new song just won't do. When the soul has been driven underground—the light of day disappearing into silent darkness, fresh breezes yielding to damp stillness—something within us longs for something deeper, something older.

It's not that new songs can't have depth. Some certainly have all the richness of the songs from our past—perhaps even more. It's just that the new song hasn't been around long enough to make its way deeply into our hearts. The songs we want sung when we're in pain are the songs that have been around long enough to become trusted friends.

Meanwhile, besides the old songs, I was getting reacquainted with another friend: the Old Testament character Job. I had read, studied, and preached on this man and his crisis before, but now I read his story with new interest.

The very fact that I was reading at all was encouraging. Throughout my ICU and hospital stay, I had not been able to read anything more than the notes on the white board. Now my mind and eyes were able to focus long enough to read at least a paragraph or two.

Family members read some of my favorite passages to me. I appreciated and benefited from these moments. But as I began to read for myself, the first place I turned was to Job. I was hungry—almost desperate—to understand his story.

Since my reading ability was limited—and since I already knew that God wasn't impressed with the answers given by Job's friends—I limited my reading to Job's statements. I skipped all the arguments raised by the other men so that I could focus on the wrestlings of a man in crisis.

*What was going on in the heart and mind of this man who had suffered so greatly? What questions was he asking? What was his attitude toward God?*

I felt that I had lost my bearings to some degree during the mind-numbing weeks in ICU. As I tried to re-engage my mind with solid thinking, I felt a need for someone to help guide me.

Job proved to be a worthy friend.

As I opened his story, I knew that Job's trial was far greater than mine. He lost his children and his wealth, his dignity and his health. A righteous and once prominent man now sits among the ashes—sooty reminders of his massive losses—scraping the puss from his oozing sores while his wife verbally punishes him with her ridicule, "Are you still holding on to your integrity? Curse God and die!" (Job 2:9).

Nice lady. Great support.

I shouldn't be too hard on Mrs. Job, though. She was in deep, deep pain as well. Yet, sadly, some people's pain becomes a poison that ruins their own souls and spills onto others.

Later I would thank Joanna for being so gracious to me through my trial. She loved me, stood by me, nursed me, supported me, cared for me, prayed with me, believed in me, and believed for me. Day after day she had been everything that Mrs. Job failed to be. In classic Joanna style, she downplayed my compliment and her role as she said, "I'd rather be a nurse than a widow."

Mrs. Job, at least according to her words, would have preferred widowhood.

Meanwhile, Job scrapes his body and wrestles with his thoughts. His friends are at their best when they sit with him in silence. His wife is never heard from again in the text. His God will show up on the scene, but not until many chapters later.

As I read snippets of Job's story each day, my mind wasn't processing thoughts in a succinct and cohesive enough manner to clearly articulate these things at the time; but my soul was finding comfort from Job's story. Later I would summarize my findings from Job as follows:

1. It is possible to be righteous and to grieve. Some forms of Christianity seem to downplay the importance of grief. Job's story teaches me that it is okay to despise my current situation...at least for a season. Spirituality does not require immediate and automatic acceptance of life's losses. With time, maturation, and assistance from the Holy Spirit, I'll eventually be able to join the New Testament author and "consider it pure joy" when I face trials of many kinds (James 1:2). But, in the meantime, I take solace from Job's words:

   "For sighing comes to me instead of food; my groans pour out like water. I have no peace, no quietness; I have no rest, but only turmoil" (Job 3:24, 26).

   Permission to be honest has been granted. Permission to grieve has as well.

   Passages that once felt heavy—even depressing—now have become a gift to me. Job reaches such discouragement that he wishes he had never even been born. I thank him—or whoever it was—that penned and preserved his powerful words...words that I would have felt guilty saying had someone before me not dared to utter them.

"Why did I not perish at birth, and die as I came from the womb?" (3:11).

2. It is possible to be righteous and yet suffer. Not all evil that befalls us is the direct result of our own sin.

3. It is possible for God to be good while allowing seasons of difficulty—even heart-crushing pain—to enter our lives. My current circumstances are not the test of God's character. My faith in His goodness must not be undermined by my current trial.

4. It is possible to take our grief too far.

I appreciated Job's honesty:

"I loathe my very life; therefore I will give free rein to my complaint and speak out in the bitterness of my soul" (10:1).

Yet, I wondered, *Doesn't there have to be a limit somewhere? I can grieve my loss and vent my frustration, but where is the line that I should not cross?*

I found it plainly detailed in Job's story, twice:

"In all this, Job did not sin by charging God with wrongdoing" (1:22).

"'Shall we accept good from God, and not trouble?' In all this, Job did not sin in what he said" (2:10).

*Somehow, in the midst of my honest wrestling and angry emotion, I must learn from Job's example and stop short of finding fault with God. He is good. He can be trusted...even when I don't understand or appreciate what He is up to.*

5. It is possible for our faith to be rebuilt in adversity. Devastating events strip our faith down to its naked form. After what I assume to be weeks of distress, Job's grief begins to unleash his anger. I hear the frustration and passion rising in his voice. At a climactic moment, with teeth-gritted, fist-pounding determination Job shouts:

"Though he slay me, yet will I hope in him" (13:15).

I hear Job saying to God, "I've got nothing left but the last gasps of life. I'm ruined! But, I'm not going to stop clinging to you. You are my only hope and if you take away the final thing I have left—my life—I'll still keep clinging to you! You're not getting rid of me, because I've got nowhere else to go but you!"

Job, in truth, had become my friend...and mentor.

# GOD-TIMING

Even though I was beginning to read again, I still had reason to fear that I had lost some of my mental capacity. It seemed that days of unconsciousness, weeks of high levels of strong medications, and events of low levels of oxygen made for a dangerous combination. My mental condition had become a continuous cause for prayer by those closest to me.

While in rehab, I became very aware that I did have short-term memory loss. By evening I couldn't tell you what I had done earlier in the day. I hoped this was just a passing condition, but I also had reason to believe I had suffered long-term memory loss.

Just when I feared it the most, God gave me a very thoughtful gift. In the night, I distinctly remembered being a three-year-old boy, and spending some time on a farm. I remembered the farmer, his wife, his dog—a collie—and a delightful feeling of being loved and happy. I was deeply encouraged by the memory. Not only was it a pleasant distraction from my physical discomfort, it was hope-giving: If I could recall some of my earliest childhood experiences, perhaps my long-term memory was okay after all.

I was curious though, *Why had I stayed with that family in the first place?*

I asked my sister the next morning if she remembered the event. She had fond memories of the family, Chet, Pauline, and their children, but didn't know why I had stayed there as a boy. It wasn't a big deal that I find out the answer, but I was curious.

That very day in the mail I received a letter from the now ninety-year-old farmer's wife. It was only the second communication we had shared since childhood. From her nursing home in Iowa, Pauline had heard of my illness and wanted to let me know that she was praying for me. In the course of her letter she explained to me what a pleasure it was to have me stay at their home so many years ago when my parents were attending a conference and needed a place for me to stay for a week.

I laughed as I read the letter.

Some people attribute such events to "coincidence." I choose to see them differently. Pauline had written a letter answering my question before I even asked it, and her letter arrived precisely on the day I became curious about the answer. It wasn't just a sweet letter from an old friend; it was a sweet reassurance from God Himself.

One of the most powerful ways God reveals His sovereignty is through timing. He could do what He does any moment He chooses. But there are instances when He—pardon the expression—"shows off" a little. Some of His acts are done at such a time that we have assurance that they are His doing.

It was a tiny incident: a memory, a question, a letter. Yet, for me it was reassurance that not only had I not lost my memory, but something else was going on as well: God was quietly working behind the scenes orchestrating events on my behalf.

It wasn't the only time at rehab that I would benefit from this conviction that God was expressing His sovereignty through timing.

I was entering my eleventh week of hospitalization. Throughout the time I had heard reports of how the church was doing and hadn't experienced a moment of worry about it. In God's kindness—and again, perfect timing—a solid and godly leadership team was in place at the church. Every key staff position was filled by someone in whom I had confidence. They were well-suited for their roles. In my absence, they had stepped up their leadership another notch and the church was effectively moving forward. Sure, they may have missed me as a person, but the team was functioning very well without me.

Yet, I knew there was an elephant in the room. No one had said a word to me, but I could feel it: *John, you've been out for a while. We've missed you, but we've got to get on with the work of the church. It's pretty obvious that you are still weak and sick and, therefore, not able to lead at this time. What should we do?*

I asked to meet with Robb, our highly trusted executive pastor. I explained to him, "It's time for me to take a leave of absence and turn the leadership over to someone else. It looks like recovery is going to take a while and I think it puts the church in an awkward position if we don't appoint someone else in my place for a season."

Robb didn't even try to hide the sigh of relief that flowed out of him. In his kindness, he hadn't wanted to raise the issue, but he was deeply grateful that I did.

A meeting of our leadership was called. Then due to scheduling issues, it had to be cancelled and rescheduled. Finally, about a dozen of us gathered in the rehab center's conference room. I tried to affirm them as a team and as individuals, and then shared with them my decision. I was stepping aside. One of our preaching team members and my wheelchair racing friend, Steve, would lead the way for this season.

"I've enjoyed being the quarterback of this team, but now I'm on the disabled list. I'll be cheering you on from the sidelines."

It was an emotional moment. I cried. I wasn't alone.

I prayed a commissioning prayer for Steve. Then, with more tears in my eyes, I asked him to take good care of the bride—Christ's church. He assured me that he would. With that, I handed him a football as a symbolic gesture of handing over the leadership.

It never crossed my mind that I wouldn't get the football back, but in my heart I sensed a release. I didn't say anything about it at the moment, but simultaneous to the hand-off of the football, my heart was handing-off something as well.

Joanna wheeled me back to my room. My emotions were too stirred and mind too busy to sleep, so she reached for the stack of cards and letters that had come in that day's mail. In it was an encouraging card from Sharon, the former executive assistant to the senior pastor. We had never worked together as she retired before I came to the church, yet I deeply appreciated her and continued to benefit from her unassigned role as "church historian." If you need a date or name of some significant moment or person in the church's eighty-year history, Sharon is the person to talk to.

In her letter, she thanked me for my service to the church and briefly reminisced about the day I had first been called—by God and the church leadership—to serve as lead pastor.

I remembered the event so clearly. The governing board had invited our whole family to again visit the church. The board and I already had been in conversation for over a year and half by this time. I had spoken as a guest preacher. I had met many leaders and been through many interviews. But I was still uncertain. I wanted to have a sense of "call." I didn't know how it would come, but I wanted God to speak into this in some way.

Seated in the middle section of the balcony during a Sunday morning service, I looked around at the congregation and prayed one more time for God's guidance in this matter…something I had done many times for many months.

Suddenly words "landed" on my heart. I didn't hear anything with my ears, but the message was unmistakable, "I'm giving you my bride, my most precious possession. Take good care of her."

I wept.

I wept because, like a dam breaking, I now had clarity and calling. I knew what God wanted me to do and I was pleased to do it. It was a pleasant calling. It was a good church. I would be their pastor.

But I wept for a greater reason. Beyond the words themselves, for a passing moment I sensed the heart of Christ Himself for His people. The sweet, tender love of the Groom for His bride was exquisitely beautiful. It was as if Jesus was weeping tears of love through me.

I would not only seek to pastor the church, but I would seek to love her with Christ's love. So, it was no surprise when a few hours later, as the church leadership met, that they issued the official call to come and serve among them. I immediately accepted.

In her letter, Sharon reminded me of these events and, in good historian style, noted the date that they had taken place. To my amazement, I had just stepped down from leadership seven years to the day that I had been first called.

Again, some may see this as mere "coincidence." For me, it was another whispered confirmation.

God was up to something. I was part of a bigger plan. I couldn't see where it was heading, but I wasn't walking this journey alone. If He was interested enough to orchestrate the hand-off of my leadership seven years to the day from my initial call, He wasn't absent from this story.

There were major parts of the story line that I didn't like, but I couldn't deny that He was in it.

# HOME

The staff at the rehabilitation center gave me a choice.

After almost three weeks under their excellent care, I was—in their determination—strong enough to go home. My health insurance authorized a longer stay, but if I thought I was ready, the staff was willing to release me.

I chose the "early out" option. However, this kicked in a series of questions we had never before faced. The staff wisely helped us think them through one-by-one:

- Would I be able to get up the stairs into my house? Yes, but only with assistance.
- Would I be able to get into bed? Yes, but only in the main floor guest bedroom. I wasn't ready for the full flight of stairs to get to our master bedroom.
- Would we be able to handle the medications and tube feeding process? Yes, Joanna was more than capable and willing to assist me.
- Would I be able to use the toilet and shower? No. We would need to have some handicap accessories installed immediately.

The conversation started to make me nervous.

*What if I have to use the toilet and Joanna isn't around? Where do you buy a walker or those handle bars to put on the toilet seat? Will I be able to function without the aid of nurses around me all the time? What if I have a setback, will I end right back up in one of these places?*

Worry was nothing new for me. I wasn't immune from the anxiety germ that can infect the heart, robbing it of peace. But, usually my anxiety had centered on bigger issues or major events. Now my apprehension seemed to rise to new levels. I felt nervous tension over these seemingly small details.

For over two months I had been in the care of others. We were soon to be on our own. Could we do this?

To complicate matters, a friend assured us he'd take care of some of these details; but after he left the rehab room, he must have forgotten because we never heard from him again on the matter. In all fairness, this experience was very rare during my crisis. Countless people came through for us with all kinds of help. However, at this key moment, as we made the preparations for independent living, we were on our own.

His oversight—small though it was—served as a good reminder to me that people who have suffered a physical setback, find themselves in a unique place of vulnerability. I was now unable to take care of these matters on my own and, as I've mentioned, I was experiencing an unfamiliar anxiety. Driving to a store, picking up a few items, driving home, carrying them up the stairs and installing them in my house was something I would have once done with ease. Now I was completely dependent. My thoughts were torn:

*How could my friend let us down like that? Did I misunderstand something? I was sure he said he'd take care of it. But, I've probably let down my share of people through the years. I never understood how vulnerable someone could feel.*

The specific issues still weren't settled, but with my eagerness to live outside of hospital walls growing by the hour, on a wet Saturday in January we were officially released. With a box of medical supplies, a wheelchair, and enough feeding tube formula to sustain me until our home shipment arrived, the nursing staff loaded me into the passenger seat of our van. I was a free man—at least as free as someone can be whose daily life is dependent on others.

My family hadn't had lunch yet. The Wendy's Drive-Thru sign lured them in. Their food smelled wonderful as it wafted through the van. They ate as we made our way to our next stop: Walmart. I stayed in the van while they shopped. Sitting before me in the beverage holder was a small Wendy's Frosty.

It called to me. It beckoned me. It spoke my language. It insisted that I give it a try.

*The therapists were just being extra cautious. How could a guy not be able to swallow something so soft, smooth, and creamy?*

I reached for the spoon and took a modest bite. I wouldn't be greedy about it, but surely I could enjoy it carefully. The burst of flavor and delightful coolness sent all those mysterious triggers to my brain telling me that this was heavenly.

*Oh, wow.*

That's when it turned ugly. As the coolness melted, my mouth and tongue couldn't control it. It slipped down into my throat...my limp, motionless throat. My windpipe was the only open hole the slithering substance could find. I got the van door open just in time as I coughed, sputtered, spat, and drooled my failed efforts onto the parking lot.

The lesson was harsh but quickly learned. I wouldn't try to sneak a bite again for a long time.

*Those therapists must have known what they were doing.*

Eventually, the family returned. Joanna had found a kit that transforms a typical toilet into one that made it more usable for me. Nifty. One less reason to be nervous.

Next we found our way to Big 5 Sporting Goods. At rehab, they had started me on a good regime of physical therapy and I was going to continue it the best I could. I just needed some small dumbbells—one, three, and five pounds. My family wheeled me inside and I spotted a man from our church. We knew each other well, had shared some significant conversations together, and I even had the privilege of performing his wedding ceremony a year earlier.

"Randall," I called out in my raspy voice, some of the air escaping out of the taped hole in my throat.

Randall turned and looked at me, figured he had misunderstood, and walked farther down the aisle.

"Randall!" I tried again.

Confused, he turned around and walked toward me. It wasn't until he came within two steps of me that his look of confusion gave way to delighted surprise, "Pastor!"

He apologized for not recognizing me. The last time he had seen me—just days before my illness began—I weighed a healthy 190 pounds. Now my six-foot-one inch frame slumped in my wheelchair weighing a scrawny 140.

In many other ways I had changed as well. My facial muscles had been decimated and I no longer had a smile or my normal facial expressions. The fascinating subtleties that give a face unique expression were gone. My hair had rapidly grayed and turned to a wiry mess. My voice was weak and barely recognizable. Joanna would privately wonder during this season, *How could a person appear to have aged so rapidly? He looks eighty years old!*

Gratefully, she never said this to me, but I had access to a mirror. I knew how dramatically I had changed. So I wasn't surprised when Randall couldn't identify me. I was just glad to be back in a normal environment, seeing a friend outside of a hospital setting.

This wasn't the only time I'd have the odd experience of not being recognized. At a clinic a few weeks later, I said "hello" from my wheelchair to a family walking past. In the last four years I had been in their home a dozen times. They knew me well. As I greeted them, they looked at me without recognition and kept walking.

Another time, in the same clinic, I sat waiting for Joanna to get the van. Standing right next to me were two women from our church. I sat and listened—in plain sight, almost close enough to touch them—while they talked:

"Have you heard how Pastor John is doing?"

"I know he's out of rehab and is home now."

"Did they ever diagnose his condition?"

On the conversation about me went. I felt almost energy-less that day, so I didn't make the effort to let them know I was right there. At the same time, I will confess, I found a twisted pleasure—like Tom Sawyer watching his own funeral—hearing what others were saying about me.

I knew I wasn't forgotten. I knew people cared. But I also knew that I had come home a completely different person than when I had been taken away in the ambulance a few months earlier.

Getting home gave me a sense of relief. I enjoyed feeling like a *family* again. I appreciated that my wife and children had visited me so often in the hospital, but now I didn't have to be "visited." I was just one of them again. Besides, the world's greatest "nurse"—Joanna—was completely mine. Although she never had a day of nurse's training, her God-given gifts and heart for me made her well-suited for the role.

I also appreciated *quiet*. Hospitals are not only a constant bustle of activity but a continual cacophony of sounds. The activity is essential and the sounds all have their purpose—alarms warning, intercoms directing, machines operating, staff discussing—but the incessant nature of it all wore on me.

I never saw the source of the most difficult sounds I heard. For about four days in rehab, I was roomed across the hall from a person—I was told she was a young woman—who evidently had periods of excruciating pain. Her sighs and groans would turn to wails...and became a solemn gift to me. I hated my condition, but another soul within just a few yards of me, was in a battle far more difficult.

It is human nature to compare ourselves with others. This often leads us to negative places. But, in this instance, her terribly difficult situation reminded me that I could have it so much worse. Gratitude was hard to come by during those days, but her story rescued me from becoming altogether ungrateful.

Now I was in the quiet of my home with my family. The early nervousness of whether we could handle everything was alleviated by the presence of visiting home health care professionals. Our mailbox overflowed with cards from family, friends, acquaintances, and people we had never met but who had heard our story and wanted to express their support. It was obvious that we weren't on this journey alone.

I was hopeful—and had good reason to be—that I was on a solid path of healing. I had hit bottom, and "bottom" was lower than I knew possible, but I was coming back. God rescued me from death and was raising me up. Confidence that I would be back to my old self in good time sustained me.

As I've already said, one of God's gifts to us is that we do not know the future. He is strong enough to know what is coming. We are not. He can see a great day on the horizon, but His foreknowledge does not spoil His joy when the great day arrives. He can see a horrible day coming without being defeated, discouraged, or distressed by it. We are not so strong.

Some of our hope—perhaps even most of our hope—is actually based on our ignorance. It must be this way for humans.

Had I known in advance what the next year would be like for me, it would have robbed what little strength I did have to face it. Instead, I was ignorant and optimistic.

Meanwhile, I had plenty going on to occupy my thoughts and time.

# BREAKING NEW GROUND

One of the odd complications I suffered was a biopsy-gone-bad.

The two inch incision the surgeon made on my left thigh to remove a muscle had healed nicely, although I was frustrated that the biopsy was inconclusive.

*You mean they cut open my leg and didn't learn anything from it?*

The process, therefore, seemed quite useless but at least it was uneventful. However, the second biopsy—this time from the thigh of my right leg—while being equally inconclusive, became a significantly more complex event.

During the weeks in ICU when I retained the seventy pounds of fluid, my body had swollen from face to feet. This created havoc with the newest wound inflicted by the surgeon's knife. By the time I was in rehab, the wound had not healed at all, but had actually worsened. Twice a day, a nurse gently stuffed over a yard of sterile gauze into the hole in my leg.

I remember thinking *I didn't know they made Q-Tips that long.*

The staff was concerned that my skin would heal over before all the layers of flesh underneath properly healed. In order to aid the healing, an extra long Q-Tip was used to poke the gauze into the open nooks and crannies of what had been an ultra-marathon running leg. I think they called the problem "tunneling." Evidently abscesses formed between and under the muscles where puss could flourish. This all sounded unpleasant enough, but then I was told that the bacteria in the puss could eat away at good flesh. I didn't complain when they cleaned the site.

One day, as a rehab doctor removed the day-old gauze, he let out a yell, "Aach! What's that?!"

I always tried to watch these procedures—it was *my* body they were working on, after all—and this one was the best. I made a veteran doctor scream. Cool.

Plopped onto my leg was something that looked like a chicken gizzard. A mass of flesh, disconnected from anything else, came out with the gauze. It caught the doctor, nurse, and me by surprise. We all just stared at it for a few moments.

They sent the mass off for testing and the report came back—in my laymen's terms—identifying it as "miscellaneous dead flesh."

Then there was the day of the HAZMAT suits. Again, I'm using non-medical terms as I describe this, but they had evidence to believe that I had contracted a really bad virus in my wound…one of those way-too-hard-to-get-rid-of and way-too-easy-to-give-to-someone-else kinds of viruses that are known to lurk around hospitals. The result was that anyone entering my room during this scare had to be fully robed and wear a face mask. And, any nurse attending to the wound had to be completely covered, including a face shield. There's nothing quite like being alone in a hospital room at night and having a nurse come through your door looking like she's preparing to deal with a nuclear disaster.

With this background, Joanna was nervous about being the nurse caring for my wound at home. I assured her that I could handle it myself. My rehab nurses—great people that they were—had let me pull out and re-stuff the gauze myself a couple times. It felt weird, but was amazingly painless. We'd be fine.

However, when the medical staff suggested that yet another surgery be done to open the wound further so that a uniform healing could take place, Joanna jumped at the idea. I offered a few objections, but they didn't carry as much weight as the advice of the professionals.

So, the "highlight" of my first week at home was to go right back to the hospital for outpatient surgery. I was awake for the procedure, although I didn't get to watch this one. That was okay, though. The smell of my own flesh being burned away—I think I heard the surgeon say something about "cauterizing the capillaries"—was sensory experience enough for me. When he was done, I asked if I could look. I gasped when I saw it. It's not every day you get a good look inside yourself. The opening in my leg was now four inches long and three inches wide...the center portion exposing my thigh muscle itself.

To aid a clean and uniform healing, I was given a "wound vacuum"—a small pack continuously attached to the surgery site via a hose, sponge, and an amazing air-tight tape. I didn't even know such inventions existed, and suddenly one became my 24/7 companion to keep the wound properly draining and to aid cell growth. The best part was that the vacuum came with Nora, a home health care nurse. She would not only replace the wound dressing and care for the vacuum three times a week; she would seek to care for my whole person: body, soul, and spirit.

Meanwhile, I became "attached" to something else: a blog. During my hospitalization, Robb, the church executive pastor, had steadily posted updates on our church website. His efforts were much appreciated by our family and were an effective means of keeping the information current, the rumor mill down, and the prayers going up.

Once I returned home, Robb suggested that I might want to write these updates myself. I accepted the challenge, primarily because I thought it would be a good way to communicate with the thousands of people who had prayed, sent cards, e-mailed, and were genuinely concerned. There was no way I could communicate with all of them individually.

My intent was to write an update every few days. Sometimes I would give the latest on my health condition, but I also intended to use the opportunity to explore what was going on in my heart during this mind-boggling journey. The discipline of writing had often helped me sort out my thoughts in the past. I sensed it would be a good practice for me during my recovery. I hoped—and prayed—that these thoughts would have value for others as well.

When I accepted the hand-off from Robb, I figured it was a good idea. I had no clue just how beneficial this would become for me. Much of my own soul health and healing would arise from the interactions started by the blog.

I found it comical: *I've rarely ever even read a blog. Here I am writing one!*

I found it therapeutic: *I never would have had the discipline to put my thoughts into print if I didn't have a commitment to communicate with others.*

I found it communal: *These people that read my blog are truly tracking with my story. Amazing. There's a world full of other things out there they could be reading. They must truly care.*

I continue to write the blog to this day, grateful for the community that continues to walk this journey with me.

I was even more excited about another opportunity to reconnect with people. After years of planning, the much awaited day had come. As my second week home from rehab ended, our church celebrated the Ground-breaking Ceremony for Broadway Commons, our new community center.

A temporary stage was set up on the parking lot. A couple men helped me up onto the platform as the band played with energy,

*Greater things are still to be done in this city.*

As the songs rang on and the crowd gathered, I felt something that had been in short supply lately: joy. It was a fulfilling and satisfying mo-ment. Not only was the church continuing to move forward with plans that I believed to be significant and city-impacting, but I was back among people I loved.

Tears immediately filled my eyes as I saw so many faces I hadn't seen in months. They had prayed me through my crisis and their joy matched mine as our eyes met. In God's kindness, the light rain stopped and the sun broke through. Even more amazing was that each speaker—our city mayor, our denominational president and yours truly—kept their remarks to less than five minutes each.

I then prayed one of the shortest public prayers I have ever prayed,

"Lord, in this place may tens of thousands of people experience the love of Christ so that many may come to know you as Savior, Leader, Lord, and Friend."

Fifty shovels were waiting, the band filled the parking lot with sounds of celebration and the entire congregation was invited to participate. I was able to get a couple digs in myself. We thrust our shovels into the soil as if to say,

"We're not going to be stopped. God has called us to do a good work in this city. Church, community and commerce will come to-

---

gether in this place for the common good. We might have setbacks, but we're moving forward. Greater things *are* yet to come. Greater works *are* still to be done and we have a part in it."

Cameras flashed. Hugs abounded. Tears flowed. I left almost two hours later exhilarated and exhausted. It had been a memorable day and I fully assumed that I'd soon be well enough to lead the church again.

# A STACK OF REMINDERS

My first hints of post-hospital discouragement started to show up not too many days after the Groundbreaking Ceremony.

As the home health care service delivered their second shipment of formula for my feeding tube, reality started to settle in. The delivery truck brought the formula eight or nine cases at a time. There they sat, stacked high on our kitchen counter. Each case carried twenty-four cans—enough for three days. Thanks to an efficient system, another shipment would arrive in a few more weeks. The soy bean and oat based "calorically dense liquid medical food" kept me alive. I grew accustomed to burps that tasted like I'd been grazing in the open field.

The stacks became symbolic...steady reminders that no one in the medical profession expected my condition to improve rapidly. I heard words like *long, slow, process, wait, patience,* and *eventually* more times than I could count. I wasn't discounting the fact that God could do a healing work in a moment's time, but I recognized that He appeared to be choosing the path of healing that required a fair amount of patience and participation on my part. I was assigned a list of exercises to strengthen my mouth, tongue, face, neck, and throat muscles. *Long* and *slow* were definitely appropriate words.

During this time one of my sisters sent me a warm letter which included verses by which she had put my name in her Bible,

"Yet I am confident I will see the LORD's goodness while I am here in the land of the living. Wait patiently for the LORD. Be brave and courageous. Yes, wait patiently for the LORD" (Psalm 27:13-14 NLT).

For the first time I noticed courage and bravery linked with patience. I could imagine David talking to himself saying, "Pull it together, man. Be brave and hang in there. God will come through in His own time, but meanwhile you have to show some courage."

My soul was unable to really feel the encouragement, but at least my head was able to grasp the concept this passage taught. In the passage of life in which I found myself, courage was necessary for patience to thrive. Fear kept rising up, telling me that I'd never improve. Discouragement would tag along like a kid brother pestering me that my efforts were worthless.

*Why even try?* An inner voice nagged.

It takes a unique type of courage to persevere when no signs of progress emerge. Yet, the stack on my counter testified that if I ever wanted to eat a pizza again, I didn't have much choice.

# PART TWO

How long, O LORD? Will you forget me forever?
How long will you hide your face from me?
How long must I wrestle with my thoughts
And every day have sorrow in my heart?
How long will my enemy triumph over me?

All my longings lie open before you, O Lord;
My sighing is not hidden from you.

The LORD will fulfill his purpose for me;
Your love, O LORD, endures forever—
Do not abandon the works of your hands.

*Psalm 13:1-2; 38:9; 138:8*

# SEQUESTERED

Our primary connection to the world outside of our house was through the steady stream of cards, emails, and blog comments that loving people continued to send to us. We were stunned by the fact that people we hadn't seen in years would remember us at this time with their prayers and verbal blessings. Occasionally a check would be enclosed as well. Incredible.

Seeing my continual need to spit, two thoughtful women in the church gave me two bundles of spit rags. Absorbent and washable, they proved to be very helpful and saved us many dollars in paper towels. One bundle of them came scripted with carefully selected scripture verses such as Joshua 1:9. *(The graphic on the cover of this book is from this actual rag.)*

I found myself saying it many times through the months that followed, "The church—the body of Christ—is amazing...when she is functioning as Christ intends."

On one memorable day, in a small stack of cards, we received the same "word" from a few significant voices in our lives. A husband and wife in Oregon and a woman in Washington—who have never met and know nothing about each other—wrote us messages that arrived on the same day. In recent years, God had used each of these mature Christians to speak insightful and even prophetic words into our lives. Now, in their correspondence to us, they both said that I was being "sequestered" for a season. This was of God's doing. I shouldn't resist it, but accept that this was for a good purpose.

The word couldn't have been more specific or timely. I was stunned that these godly voices were in agreement both in message and timing. They not only had the same general message for me, they had used the very same and rarely used word. I knew I could go through long stretches of my life and not encounter the word "sequestered" and here I'd received it twice in a day.

I received it as from the Lord and knew it to be accurate...but that doesn't mean I liked it.

I was accustomed to a very active and people-filled life. Our local church would see more than 4,000 people on our campus each week. Our staff of fifty or more was always bustling with dreams, prayers, plans, questions, concerns, tears, and laughter. My weeks were filled with meetings, conversations, lunches, decision-making, preaching, and everywhere I turned: more people.

I was active and loved to be active. I'd often commute to work on my bicycle, run a half-dozen miles after work or try to talk one of my sons into hitting a tennis ball with me. Every summer was another opportunity to climb one more mountain, run a few more races, catch a few more fish, hike a few more trails, mow more grass, and make more memories. I had the goal of riding my bike 10,000 miles before I turned fifty and was on track to meet my goal.

Suddenly this active, people-filled life came to a halt. My life was now primarily lived in 1,000 square feet...a few rooms of our house. The primary trail I traveled was with my walker between my bed and recliner. Other than our home health care professionals and a few faithful friends, most of our days were spent alone.

The church, in their gracious efforts to protect me, ceased to bring to me any leadership issues. My voice was almost unintelligible on the phone. I didn't have the energy to go anywhere, except to an occasional doctor's visit and to church once a week.

"Sequestered" became more than a concept. It was an accurate description of my life.

Through the years I had preached on the theme of waiting. Using stories of the Old Testament characters, Moses, Joseph, and David, I would teach, "God does some of His best work in waiting rooms. God has been known to take a leader and set him aside for a season. What might feel like wasted years is actually part of His training in the life of the leader. He's developing the man before He releases him to accomplish His plan."

I was now living out my own sermon and, as I said, I didn't like it.

When our son, Drew, was just three-years-old we moved from Minnesota to Colorado. In the first few days after our move, Drew curled up on the carpet and cried, "I want my old house back."

Now here I was, a forty-nine-year-old guy, curled up in bed crying, "I want my old life back."

Crying was actually something Joanna encouraged from me. I was ashamed of it, but she gently counseled me that it was healthy.

It happened more than once. We were on our way to another medical appointment, she in the driver's seat and I in the passenger's. We would pass a few joggers on the side of the road. I would watch their every step and let out a deep sigh. Joanna would gently say, "It's okay to grieve."

She gave me permission to let my heart feel what it was feeling. My "buck up and be tough" mindset scolded me at those moments for my emotions. But Joanna kept insisting that they were valid. "It's okay to cry. You need to grieve."

Wise words. Wise woman.

# LIFE AS CAREGIVER
## FROM JOANNA'S PERSPECTIVE

As the reality of our new life situation dawned on me, I felt shell-shocked. My strong confident husband of the previous fall was suddenly too weak to brush his own teeth or comb his hair. He came out of rehab looking like an eighty-year-old man. He had lost fifty pounds of muscle weight. I cried inside the first time I saw him without a shirt. He looked like pictures I had seen of concentration camp victims with every rib visible under a thin layer of skin. The muscles in his face had been so weakened that he was unable to truly smile or form words correctly. His soft palette didn't completely close, giving his voice a strong nasal quality. His hair had turned almost completely gray. I had no idea a body could change that drastically in three months time. My heart ached for his suffering and brokenness. I was compelled to try to make him as comfortable as I possibly could.

Our once relatively full, happy days became a surreal series of endless trips to clinics, doctors' offices, and pharmacies. I grieved for Drew when he was at home and wished our house didn't seem so clouded by sadness. It was terribly hard for both Drew and I to try to eat quietly in the kitchen knowing John was in the other room grieving his inability to join in.

It didn't help that I was very inexperienced and insecure in dealing with medical issues. And, I wasn't the only one who was confused. A sister-in-law wisely explained to me that if John had had a heart attack, the medical community could tell me what to expect and when to expect it. But this was so unknown there was no history to glean from.

Underlying these insecurities was the ubiquitous fear that John would regress or even die in my care. He seemed so fragile. I'd often wake up in the night and reach over in bed to see if he was still breathing.

In spite of this, as I look back at those long, dark days, I'm struck by how often Jesus showed up in small, yet very personal ways. I found myself fascinated by Genesis 39:20b-21 that says, "But while Joseph was there in the prison, the LORD was with him; he showed him kindness and granted him favor...." Obviously Joseph's desire must have been for God to get him out of prison, but even as God was denying that request, He was showing up, showing kindness, and granting favor. I knew that to be true for us as well.

One sweet example of this was our home health care nurse, Nora. She came three times a week to change John's wound vacuum system. In her positive hope-giving way, she often changed our mood and outlook as well. She is a believer, and we both grew to sincerely look forward to her visits.

Another bright spot was the spontaneous prayer gatherings our boys and their friends often formed in our living room for their Dad. It was so encouraging to listen to these young adults worship God with their voices and guitars and pray with faith for John's healing. Though he wasn't aware of any physical healing during these times, soul healing was definitely taking place.

One day on our way to yet another doctor's appointment, I was especially aware of Jesus' presence. As I helped John maneuver his way down a few short steps on our walk to the car, the wheel of his walker caught on the concrete. I realized slowly what had happened, but I was too late and too weak to catch him as he fell away from me. His head landed right between two huge landscaping rocks. An inch either way and he would have been seriously injured. But other than some minor scrapes and frustration, he was fine.

As I reflect on this era, the most obvious emotions I felt were pain and loss for both John and myself. Surprisingly, however, underneath those was a new sense of purpose and personal fulfillment. In our previous twenty-seven years of marriage, I always had a nagging sense of not pulling my weight in ministry as John's wife. He is highly gifted in *many* ways and though I thoroughly loved being a mother and homemaker, I had always struggled in my role as a pastor's wife. I am an introvert who avoids the spotlight at almost all cost. I sensed I had the gifts of mercy and encouragement, and used them in quiet, behind the scenes ways, but otherwise was always pretty unsure of my role in the body of Christ as a whole and specifically in our various churches.

With the release of John from rehab into my untrained "nursing" hands, my world turned upside down. Suddenly the confident man who had seemed to have such little need for my mercy or encouragement was almost completely in my care. Though a bit overwhelming at first, I was soon aware of God flooding my heart with His compassion and love for this broken man who had lost *so much* on so many levels, in such a short time. My Boston marathon-qualifying husband couldn't even walk into his own house or wash his own face. As I took care of him physically in ways I never imagined, I truly felt privileged to serve him.

So often in my life I had questioned why God had made me the way He had. I suddenly understood that *Jesus* was loving and ministering to John through my hands and voice. I experienced a deep understanding that this was why I was created, "for such a time as this." I don't believe there can be any more profound sense of fulfillment than being used by God in exactly the way He planned when He knit us together stitch by stitch.

To John's amazing credit, he could not have been sweeter or more grateful to me. He never once took his discomfort or pain out on me in bitterness or anger, but daily and consistently expressed his appreciation and love for me. I had never felt so valued or precious to him. God was quietly giving care to my deepest emotional needs, as I was busy giving care to my dear broken husband.

# STALLED

As February rolled into March and April, I was not improving physically. My muscles were not getting stronger—I found removing a lip balm lid a herculean task and moving my blankets in bed almost impossible. If I fell, which happened more than once, I was completely unable to get up without assistance. More than one therapist worked with me to strategize how I might get up on my own off the floor, but my muscles were simply too weak to do so. I still needed the walker to get around the house and the wheelchair if we went anywhere.

My lack of muscular strength wasn't the only issue. I was still attached to the wound vacuum as the opening in my leg was only slightly reduced in size. My skin was very frail, often painful to the touch and broke out in continual rashes. I spent many days itching, trying not to itch, or trying yet another skin ointment to alleviate the itch. I lived with a mild undercurrent of pain. I was anemic, mysteriously losing blood faster than my body was able to replace it. Pain randomly roamed around my muscles, unpredictable and unrelenting. My ability to swallow remained completely non-functioning.

But none of these conditions consumed my thinking as much as the fact that I was continuously experiencing something worse: I couldn't shake the overpowering sense of continual illness. The "bleh" I originally felt plummeted to new depths. I lived with an every-cell-in-my-body-is-sick-and-I-hate-it feeling.

Later, when telling my story to churches, I tried to describe my state by using a lame joke, "I felt horrible. I felt like a word I shouldn't say from this pulpit."

I could tell that my physical and speech therapists were disappointed in my lack of progress. I know I was.

In efforts to improve my speech and regain the ability to swallow, I was assigned various exercises numerous times a day. Neck lifts, mouth stretches, gargling Club Soda, tongue strengthening maneuvers and pages of hard to pronounce words—like "battle" and "beetle"—were part of my daily regime. Who knew that we have so many muscles giving movement to our face, lips, throat, and neck? The tongue itself is one of the body's most significant muscles. And it seemed that the disease ransacked every one of them.

I kept records to verify to my speech/swallow therapist that I was doing the assigned work. There were some days I didn't have the energy to do any of it, but in March alone I gargled well over 100 times. Meanwhile the physical therapist assigned various stretches and lifts for my arms and legs.

It was a sad day when I realized I couldn't therapy my way out of this problem. I hoped that if I just worked hard enough, I could beat whatever this was and rebuild myself. By April—three months into my post-hospitalization journey—I concluded it was impossible to overcome my profound muscle weakness through exercise alone.

My speech/swallow therapist informed me we were going to take a month off. Our efforts, it seemed, were only wearing me out and not evidencing any signs of progress.

Whatever had ravaged my body was still active to some degree. It was becoming increasingly clear that I needed help beyond what I or those around me had to offer.

Medically, the local rheumatologist kept prescribing different drugs. One of them made me feel horrible, caused nausea, and made my hair fall out. Another didn't seem to have any negative side effects but neither did it help. I came home from one treatment to take a nap, only to find I couldn't get warm. A surreal case of the "chills" came over me and a dozen blankets, a stocking cap, and a space heater weren't enough to warm me.

Spiritually, Joanna and I were surrounded by prayer and made ourselves available for any healing prayer opportunity. I was anointed with oil by our church elders on more than one occasion. I accepted any offer when someone wanted to pray over me. We went to a healing room ministry in another town, and received gracious attention, but no sign of divine intervention.

Privately, I kept my life-long practice of reading a portion of scripture and attempting to pray some sort of prayer every day. However, I'll confess that the scripture felt like sandpaper to my soul.

The stories of miracles and statements of promise seemed to mock me. During these months of spring, I was attempting to write a Bible study series for our church from the life of Jeremiah, but found his continual hardships wearying. Passages that once delighted my soul and gave substance to a sermon now sat silent on the page. The "sandpaper" may have been doing a good work within me, but in the meantime it was irritating...abrasive.

Going to church wasn't any easier. To alleviate the crowding of our Sunday services and to open the doors for people who had to work on Sundays, we had launched Saturday night church a few years earlier. In my weakened state, the weekend church concept became very helpful. The 5:00 Saturday service, because of the time of day and the smaller crowds, was the least difficult service for me to attend.

However, I'll confess that 4:40 on Saturday afternoon was the most difficult time of the week for Joanna and me. Every Saturday we dreaded the arrival of that moment when we'd look at each other and agree to do it all over again. Before this, I never understood Christians who regularly skipped church. Whether I was a pastor or not, I always attended because I truly wanted to.

But now I was facing something new. Nothing within me, it seemed, wanted to go to church and it was a struggle for Joanna as well.

Physically it required a fair amount of work to get me and a wheelchair out of the house, in and out of the van and into the church. What's more, I really missed leading and preaching and was jealous of those who did so instead of me. But these weren't the biggest reasons for our reluctance.

The real issue was that in our pain, we wanted to choose isolation. Emotionally, it took everything we had to face people. Regarding spiritual matters, we wanted to convince ourselves that we'd be just as well off to stay at home and read our Bibles together. We were weary. Any attempts to interact with the public—even great church people—felt as if they would drain our last ounce of strength.

Pain and isolation are dangerous companions. One supports and strengthens the other. Walls are built. Relationships, at the very time when we need them the most, dwindle. Our own thoughts—a place we spend more than enough time already—become the only thoughts we have; unless of course we take the popular alternative of numbing ourselves with hours of television.

I can't say that I got much out of the church services during this season of our lives, good though they may well have been. That whole concept—"getting something out of a service"—arises from a consumer mindset anyway. Yet, I believe that it was essential that we attended when we wanted to the least. Our worlds, already small, would have shriveled even further without this act of discipline.

Being the kind of person I am, I had to try to make some sense of why I was going to church in spite of my lack of desire. During my least favorite season to attend church, I recorded some reasons why I kept going anyway:

Looking back over the last few months, I realize that by attending church...

...I think thoughts I would not otherwise think

...I hear truths I would not otherwise hear

...I sing songs I would not otherwise sing

...I meet people I would not otherwise meet

...I give offerings I may not otherwise give

...I rejoice in missions' efforts and in new followers of Jesus that I would not otherwise know about

...I receive encouragement and challenge I would not otherwise receive

...I shed tears I would not have otherwise shed

...I receive a blessing I would not otherwise have received

...I pray prayers I would not have thought to pray

...I meet God in a way I would not have met Him had I stayed home in my chair

…And, perhaps, my attendance is an encouragement or testimony to someone else.

When I'm there, I may not like every song or agree with every word spoken. But that's not the point. I may have wrestled with Him all week; but come the weekend I publically present myself again to acknowledge my allegiance to Him. Satan may have beaten me around during the week, but I'm going to show up in church again and declare Whose side I'm on.

I now understand how easy it is for people to slip out of the habit of church attendance. And I now understand even more fully the significance of the words in Hebrews admonishing us, "Let us consider how we may spur one another on toward love and good deeds. Let us not give up meeting together, as some are in the habit of doing, but let us encourage one another—and all the more as you see the Day approaching" (Hebrews 10:24-25).

No weekend, however, quite matched the difficulty of Good Friday and Easter.

# BROKEN BREAD, BROKEN SPIRIT

As a pastor, Good Friday was often a spiritually significant day for me. I loved participating in this rich remembrance as I led Good Friday services. I would participate again this year, but this time from the back row of the congregation in the wheelchair section.

I squirmed uncomfortably in my chair as I watched the worship team assemble on the platform. My body was in pain and my spirit low. Yet, the music was fabulous and my spirit was soon drawn into worship. Then came the moment of sharing together in communion. I asked Joanna to wheel me to the front, received the piece of bread and dipped it in the juice…fully knowing I had no ability to consume it. Returning to the back row, I touched the bread to my tongue, prayed a prayer and wrapped the bread in one of my ever-present spit rags.

The petrified morsel remains in my desk drawer still today as an odd symbol of my need and His provision.

On Saturday evening we attended the Easter Service. Again, the difficulty of not being able to participate from the platform was overcome by the beauty and truth of the music. A month earlier I could sing a range of six notes—cracked and weak though they were—but notes nevertheless. By Easter I lost all six. Here it was, the grandest celebration of the Christian year, and I had no voice to sing. My feeble but joyful noise had been reduced to a whisper and a mere mouthing of the words. So, much to the consternation of the three-year-old in the pew in front of me who would not stop watching me the entire hour, I whispered and mouthed my way through the service.

And, I knew I would rather have a reason to sing but no voice than have a voice and no true reason for song.

What I dreaded most was Easter Sunday itself. It would be such a stark contrast to every other Easter our family had enjoyed. I didn't want to even think about it. But, days arrive whether we are ready for them or not. I purposely slept in as late as I possibly could and then "took" my wife and Drew to a family favorite, Red Lobster. Sitting at a restaurant while others ate wasn't my favorite thing to do, but I really wanted the family to have some semblance of an Easter meal...besides, someone had given our family a gift card.

Our meal wasn't what you'd describe as joyful, but we were having a pleasant enough time when—bam! I got hit with a double-barrel-full-gusher bloody nose. I stuffed napkins up my nose, tossed the gift card for Drew to handle and asked Joanna to rush me—as much as a guy with a walker can be rushed—to the van before I made a bigger scene than I already had. I was very embarrassed as we shuffled past the Easter Sunday crowd. At the moment, it felt like more than a bloody nose. It felt like humiliation. As soon as we made it out the restaurant door, I defiled the sidewalk with globs of bloody spit. Joanna helped me into the passenger's seat of the van and went back to clean up the sidewalk mess.

Forty five minutes later we were home with the bloody situation fully under control again; but the ordeal felt like one more blow. I was angry:

*I can't take communion, I can't sing, I can't eat, I can't take my family out for a decent meal without making a scene!*

I finished the weekend by re-reading a chapter from Samuel Rutherford, a pastor in England during the 1600s. For a season he was exiled from his congregation in England by the state church. They sent him to a different part of the country and banned him from preaching. In his state of exile, he wrote numerous letters to friends which have been preserved in a book simply titled *Letters of Samuel Rutherford*.

A few months into exile he wrote of his inability to preach which he referred to as his "sad silence." On November 22, 1636, he wrote, "I have wrestled long with this sad silence. I said, what aileth Christ at my service? And my soul has been at pleading with Christ...But I will yield to Him, providing my suffering may preach more than my tongue did... In a word, I am a fool, and He is God. I will hold my peace hereafter."

His words helped bring perspective to my weekend. I could only hope that "my suffering may preach more than my tongue" had. And, I hoped that I would preach with my voice again as well.

I was attempting to keep my attitude good and my spirits up. However, it was a daily battle that I didn't always win.

On more than one occasion, the combination of my medication and feeding tube formula didn't settle well with my stomach causing me to vomit. I remember thinking, *What kind of sadistic joke is this? Why can food come up my esophagus but not go down?!*

One afternoon, as I was attempting to take a nap, the sudden urge to vomit arose. I leaned over the edge of the bed to grab a garbage can. As the retching began, I felt myself slipping out of bed and onto the floor. I tried to call out to the family, but the bedroom door was closed and my voice too weak for anyone to hear. My stomach soon settled down, but my spirit was rattled.

I felt pathetic. There I was, on the floor next to a garbage can of my vomit, without enough strength to get up or enough voice to summon someone to help me. I don't know if my proud heart has yet been fully broken through this entire journey, but if there was a definite breaking moment, this was it. An odd prayer arose within me, *God, if you allow me to preach again, I'll preach anywhere you send me.*

It wasn't a plea. I wasn't bartering with Him, "If you will heal me, then I will preach." No, it wasn't a bargain; it was a breaking.

*I want to serve you again. You decide where.*

Images of places, both humble and prestigious, came to mind.

*Anywhere, Lord.*

I heard footsteps in the hall.

"Help, please," my raspy voice pled.

"Dad?"

Drew came in through the door, gently lifted me back into bed and, unsure what to say, quietly slipped away. I felt lonely.

*What was that word again? It starts with an "s." Set aside? Isolated? Sequen…. Sequestered. That's it. Yep, that's exactly it.*

# SILENCE

The days started to drag. Never in my life had I felt how horribly long a day could be. Magnifying this feeling was the fact that one of my favorite daily diversions had been taken away from me: meals. As much as the pleasure of eating, I missed the social interaction that goes with meals. When life was "normal," food and conversation highlighted a day hundreds of times a year. Pouring formula down my tube was no substitute. It kept my body alive, but did nothing for my spirit, and did nothing to break up my day. It was merely one more reminder of my broken condition.

I tried to keep the tone of my blog as positive as I could, but by May I admitted, "I haven't been doing too well in recent days. My mind has been mush. My emotions feel like they've been run through a paper shredder. My body keeps coming up with new ways to make life unpleasant."

Through it all, I kept trying to find God. My spiritual journey over the decades had been marked by the normal ebb and flow of a personal relationship. Some days I felt close to God: enjoying sweet moments of worship, sensing that I had heard His heart for an upcoming sermon, or experiencing the freedom which allowed me to pour out my heart to Him in prayer. On other days though, my soul was too cluttered and noisy to really connect with Him. But through the decades, I never had reason to doubt that He would draw near to me again, if I just took the time to find a quiet place to "hang out" with Him...or at least found a quiet place in my heart to listen to Him.

I knew the promise, "Come near to God and he will come near to you" (James 4:8).

Through the years, I often experienced the pleasure of that promise being fulfilled.

But now, I couldn't find Him. I tried to pray, wait, read, listen, worship...do all the things that had "worked" before. Now, He seemed nowhere to be found.

Someone asked me one day, "How is it with your soul?"

"I'm just trying to not be angry at God," I answered.

My temptation to anger wasn't as much about being upset with my health crisis, although I certainly had to wrestle through that issue. During this season, my greater frustration came from His silence.

I scuffled with the words of C. S. Lewis, *God whispers to us in our pleasures, speaks to us in our conscience, but shouts in our pains: It is His megaphone to rouse a deaf world.*

I recorded my reaction to these words in an article I never made public, *With all due respect for one of the greatest writers in Christian history, I beg to differ with Dr. Lewis. I agree with him in principle. I understand his point. I assume that his statement is often true. But I must confess that this has not been my experience in my season of greatest pain.*

If God was shouting, I was completely deaf. For long months, I didn't feel like I was hearing anything from heaven. In the very time I expected to sense Him most, I experienced Him the least. If there was ever a time I felt like I needed His touch, it was now, but no touch seemed to come. Heaven's silence was the loudest thing I heard.

I had often heard of the historic Christian concept of "the dark night of the soul." Now it wasn't merely a concept. It was reality.

Meanwhile, friends wrote to me saying that they were waiting in eagerness to hear the great things God was teaching me through my death bed experience. The assumption they held, and I had previously as well, was that the harder the experience, the greater the lessons. If God shouts to us in our pain, His megaphone should have been pointed right at my ear. What glorious truths I would come forth from my crisis proclaiming!

Instead, I arose from my deathbed to find myself in a wheelchair—in body *and* spirit. I believed in God. I sought God. I loved God. I just couldn't find God. My spirit was as weak as my body.

Looking back on this time, I can now testify that this was a good season for me. Rich work was happening in the silence. God's silence does not equal His absence. His teaching is not limited to words. Maybe Lewis' comments had greater meaning than I realized: God's loudest "shout" might be complete silence. Sometimes silence can speak more "loudly" than words.

Now I can see with faith's eye that God was sitting with me during those long months—ever present, although silent. Yet, while I was enduring that season, my eyes weren't sharp enough—my faith not strong enough—to sense His presence. I couldn't see then what I see now.

I remembered a sermon my brother, Jim, had given over a decade earlier. In it he stated, "It is enough to exist for the glory of God alone."

He cited the example of wild flowers blooming on a remote mountain slope—to live and die never to be seen by a human—but to exist purely for God's glory and pleasure. When I first heard the message, I loved the simple yet powerful beauty of that truth. I even preached it myself a few times.

Now, I knew that I had to apply this truth layers deeper in my heart than I had previously imagined. My life, once a hub of activity, now stood almost silent like an abandoned building.

Day after day at my request, Joanna read to me the words of Jeremiah's lament, "It is good to wait quietly for the salvation of the LORD. It is good for a man to bear the yoke while he is young. Let him sit alone in silence, for the LORD laid it on him...Is it not from the mouth of the Most High that both calamities and good things come?" (Lamentations 3:26-28, 38).

My head heard what my heart couldn't feel, *God is in this, even in the silence, and He is good.*

Jeremiah understood what it was to be sequestered. But in the midst of his deep sadness, he still found the faith to declare, "Men are not cast off by the Lord forever. Though he brings grief, he will show compassion, so great is his unfailing love. For he does not willingly bring affliction or grief to the children of men" (Lamentations 3:31-33).

Existing for the glory of God, sitting alone in silence, sequestered—this was the path God had assigned to me.

I prayed for myself and those who were in similar life situations, "May God grant us the grace to blossom on whatever hillside He has planted us."

# THE SIGH OF SUNSET

The setting sun and evening darkness would bring a sense of relief. Another day—another long miserable day—was almost done. Two evening activities became a genuine gift to me.

As many as three times a week, a fairly new friend, Kendall, began coming to our house. He would set up a portable massage table and patiently rub my muscles. He wasn't trained in the craft, but was eager to find practical ways to assist me. He believed that massages might help me in my condition. I was reluctant at first, but soon became very grateful to him.

There is something uniquely comforting about human touch. While Joanna, Kendall, and his wife, Cathy, visited or watched a movie, I would lie on the table and sigh a thousand sighs. I don't know from a technical standpoint what was actually taking place in my body, but it was as if pains were being rubbed away and life was incrementally returning cell by cell. I was content for him to spend an entire hour just working my head, face, and neck over and over.

*Oh that feels good.*

One night Kendall brought over a special pillow that was open in the middle—it looked like a giant donut—to put around my feeding tube so that I could lay on my stomach. Brilliant. Now he could rub my back as well.

*Ahhh.*

And every night before he'd leave, he'd kneel beside me one more time and pray for complete healing. He was dogged in his determination.

The lack of evidence of any answers to his prayer didn't stop him. Each night he'd ask—he'd knock—again.

Some nights I could pray along. Other nights I struggled. On those nights, I'd just listen and try to ride piggy-back on his faith. My faith legs had given out, but was it okay to throw my weight onto his? This was a new experience for me. I'd always had my own faith. Now I was struggling.

*Is it legitimate…legal…to hold onto the faith of a friend?*

I was surprised by my own conclusion. When my faith ran out, there were others around me who still believed for me and, yes, it was valid, appropriate…legal, to hold onto their faith. It was okay that I didn't know what to think, ask, or pray at times. Others did. Night after night, Joanna was one of these faithful people as well.

I don't know that I really recognized what I was doing at the time. But later it was clear to me: *God, there were times I didn't know what to think of you. I didn't know what I believed. But people like Kendall and Joanna kept hanging onto you so I hung onto their faith. I was down to a bare thread, but their rope held strong so I clung to it.*

I've come to believe that my experience is a common one. While our own faith is being hammered, pulverized, shredded, or threatened to its very core, we have others around us who keep believing for us.

Hear me: It's okay to latch onto their faith when you seem to have little left of your own.

On many nights, when Joanna and I were alone, we fell into a second healthy habit. Since the dining room in our home wasn't being used very often, we designated a corner of it as my home "office." Our computer, loaded with some of our favorite music, sat on a small table. We turned off the lights and turned on some selected songs. Joanna sat on the floor with her back to the wall. I reclined in my padded desk chair. With a candle flickering, the powerful and soothing voices of the group *Selah*, ministered to us.

*O the deep, deep love of Jesus, vast, unmeasured, boundless, free!*
*Rolling as a mighty ocean in its fullness over me!*
*Underneath me, all around me, is the current of Thy love*
*Leading onward, leading homeward to Thy glorious rest above!*

Over and over we clicked "replay." Some nights we turned the volume up as loud as we could on our little speakers. Like waves, the voices, strings, lyrics, and Spirit flowed over us. The pure beauty of the music gave weight to the truth of the words:

> *O the deep, deep love of Jesus, spread His praise from shore to shore!*
> *How He loveth, ever loveth, changeth never, evermore!*
> *How He watches o'er His loved ones, died to call them all His own;*
> *How for them He intercedeth, watcheth o'er them from the throne!*

> *O the deep, deep love of Jesus, love of every love the best!*
> *'Tis an ocean full of blessing, 'tis a haven giving rest!*
> *O the deep, deep love of Jesus, 'tis a heaven of heavens to me;*
> *And it lifts me up to glory, for it lifts me up to Thee!*

Sometimes we'd pray together. Sometimes we'd just sit in silence until one of us were tired enough to justify going to bed. Joanna faithfully assisted me with all the necessary details to get me ready for the night: putting ointment on my red patches of skin, tending to the wound vacuum, getting my legs up onto the bed, adjusting the blankets, and gathering some clean spit rags or tearing off a dozen sheets of paper towels to be placed on each side of my pillow.

I'd close my eyes and picture another mile marker. Back in my marathon running days, I had relished the sense of accomplishment every time a mile marker was passed. Posted on the side of the road was a sign declaring that one more mile was complete and didn't have to be run again. As I passed, I'd coach myself,

> *Mile 1. Pace yourself. Don't get too excited.*
> *Mile 6. Off to a good start.*
> *Mile 13. Cool. Almost half-way.*
> *Mile 17. You can do this.*
> *Mile 18. One more down.*
> *Mile 19. Getting tough. Not quitting.*
> *Mile 20. Only 10-K left.*
> *Mile 22. You never have to run another race, but you're going to finish this one!*
> *Mile 23. This isn't supposed to be easy. If it were easy, everyone would be doing it.*

The obvious factor of a marathon is that the runner knows exactly how many miles the event will be: 26.2 for a normal marathon. Other types of events have their own distances. Sixty kilometers (about thirty-six miles) was the longest race I had run. My illness dashed my plans to run a hundred kilometer race through the mountains.

The difficulty of this marathon I was running is that I had no clue how long it would be. How many more days—miles—stretched before me? I had no way of knowing. However, I did find solace in the fact that the day I had just completed never needed to be lived again. I passed another marker. Tomorrow might look dreadfully like today, but at least it would be a new day.

Joanna would kiss me on the forehead, turn off the light, and slip out of the room to have a quiet hour to herself.

# SONGS IN THE NIGHT

Sleep was not easy to sustain for any length of time. It would happen thousands of times over the months. I settled down and sensed sleep approaching only to feel saliva pooling up in my throat with nowhere to go. Left too long, I would begin to choke on it. The normal person swallows so automatically that it is not a conscious act. But for me, it demanded that I grab yet another spit rag and spit again.

It wasn't much of a joke, but I would later try to make light of my continuous need to spit when speaking to younger audiences:

"How did your pastor die?"

"He drowned in his own saliva."

Nice.

A young-at-heart member of our church added her good-natured cheer to my attempts at humor. She had a t-shirt made for me which read, "Spit Happens."

So, it does. I don't know where she got the statistic, but my speech/swallow therapist told me that a normal person swallows a thousand times a day.

Yep. Spit happens, and it was happening a lot.

Meanwhile, God was giving me a nightly gift. The gift began during my weeks in ICU and continued well into this current season. I was being given songs in the night. I say "given" because I would wake up numerous times

---

in the night with specific songs already on my heart and mind. I hadn't consciously tried to recall them. They simply arose from within and, like Joanna and I hitting "replay" on our computer, kept repeating within me.

In ICU, for many nights, the song was one we had recently been singing at church. It was a song of declaration by Chris Tomlin that God is active and involved in this world, *Greater things are yet to come, greater things are still to be done in this city....*

During my stay at rehab, the song changed to an old Twila Paris tune, *God is in control, we believe that His children will not be forsaken....*

I often couldn't remember very many of the words, but the melody and main message of the song would play over and over in my heart.

When I got home, a new song emerged. I don't know that I had heard it more than a time or two in twenty years, but the sounds of Petra filled me each night, *Don't let your heart be hardened, Don't let your love grow cold.*

Each song seemed to carry its own timely theme. Each, a message from God:

- You appear to be on your deathbed, but I'm not done with you yet.
- There is more going on here than just some mysterious disease and a medical intervention. I'm still on my throne.
- You are struggling. I know it. Don't lose heart. You have to take responsibility for how you respond to this trial.

Then, of course, there was one night when my entire "God is speaking to me in songs" theory came into question. I had been having recurring dreams of food—usually food that I couldn't access. A hot, delicious looking pizza is on the roof. It's just waiting for someone to climb up and eat it. I scramble up a ladder. My ladder is a couple feet too short. I can't reach it. Someone else eats the pizza.

In another dream I am in charge of a dinner. We're feeding a couple hundred people. All is set. The food looks great! I'll eat, too. Suddenly masses of young people arrive—thousands. We don't have enough to feed everyone. I race throughout the convention center trying to find help. I find none. Many of us will go hungry this night.

I could tell you a dozen of these dream stories, but you get the idea: Food was on my mind.

So, I guess I shouldn't be too surprised that one night, my "song" was: *Two all beef patties, special sauce, lettuce, cheese, pickles, onions on a sesame seed bun.*

That wasn't real helpful.

Happily, another song arose and stayed with me for weeks. It was new to me. We were just beginning to sing it at church. I didn't get most of Matt Redman's lyrics right. But the theme kept beckoning and challenging:

*Oh no, you never let go. Lord, you never let go of me.*

The song reminded me that our God is a God with a long history of walking with people through dark valleys, even ones called death. He'd keep walking with me.

# WHAT GOES IN BY THE TUBE...

I became a regular with the phlebotomists at the clinic. Dr. Byrkit wanted to monitor various things, including my anemia. It seemed that I must have some internal bleeding. He expressed increasing concern that I had cancer.

Cancer. It's a word no one ever wants to hear.

This concern was elevated because of another factor. Dr. Byrkit had become convinced that I had Dermatomyositis—a disease of the autoimmune system that damages skin and muscle tissue. This diagnosis in no way explained all that had about killed me months earlier, but was the condition that now lingered in my body. He gently informed me that a significant percentage of people who battle Dermatomyositis also battle cancer.

A colonoscopy was ordered. This was the most likely place that the internal bleeding and/or cancer would be detected. For once my inability to swallow came in handy. Rather than having to actually drink the three liters of intestinal Drano to prepare for the procedure, we could simply pour it down my tube. A guy has to count his blessings wherever he can find them.

The greater blessing was that no cancer was found. And, I was soon to find another benefit of having a feeding tube.

My stomach occasionally refused to process the formula. Even though it was being fed the exact same thing every day, there were some days my stomach went on strike. Hours later I could feel that the formula sat undigested.

I know that not everyone appreciates reading these kinds of details, but to bypass these stories is to gloss over the real moments that made up this era.

One night, after Joanna helped me into bed, I knew I was going to vomit. Suddenly the thought hit me, *Wait a minute! If it went in by the tube, it can come out by the tube!*

Joanna helped me into the bathroom and I grabbed a feeding tube syringe. The medical supply company frequently sent us boxes of the two-ounce plastic tubes with our formula shipments. They came with a little plunger. The syringe fit into the feeding tube and made pouring formula into the tube easy and efficient. The plunger was provided, for a variety of reasons, but was especially helpful if the tube ever became clogged. Applying a small amount of pressure to the plunger would almost always push away the blockage and allow the tube to flow freely again.

At this moment, however, as my stomach churned and ached, the plunger became a very effective way to suction *out* of my stomach the undigested formula.

I'll spare most of the details of the smell and appearance of what I withdrew. It's enough for you to know that a few minutes later, eighteen ounces of the nastiest substance I'd ever encountered were no longer tormenting me. I washed the curdled mess down the sink, but its stench still permeated the room.

Joanna watched from a distance with concern, "I'm not sure you should be doing that! Did Nora tell you that was okay?"

I didn't know. I just knew I felt better.

Joanna decided we'd better take advantage of the twenty-four hour phone number that had been provided for us. Nurses were available around the clock to answer questions, and we hadn't yet used the service.

"My husband feels like he needs to vomit. He suctioned out a bunch of stuff from his stomach through his feeding tube. Is it okay that he did that?"

"Yes, that's fine if he takes it out," the nurse explained. "But, he has to put it back in so that the PH balance in his system doesn't get thrown off."

Joanna was still on the phone and I was still in the bathroom as she relayed to me the nurse's message.

I didn't know a thing about PH balance. I still don't. The closest thing

I know to a "PH balance" is that a good balance of Pizza Hut is about twice a month.

"Put it back in? Put it back in?!" I was incredulous.

"Tell her to put a straw in the toilet and suck her vomit back out!" I yelled.

Joanna just rolled her eyes at me and kindly thanked the nurse for her time.

"Put it back in, put it back in," I kept muttering. "You've got to be kidding."

I ignored her advice, bad patient that I am. And, it was another obvious example that I'd have to determine my own level of participation in my recovery. The medical community could advise, but couldn't be at my side every minute. There were some decisions I'd have to make.

Meanwhile, God *would be* at my side every moment, but it was up to me to decide how to respond to Him. What level of trust would I place in Him?

# FORMULAS OR FAITH?

My understanding of the ways God works was again put to the test one night in late May. The national conference of our denomination—a couple thousand believing people—were gathered in Louisville, Kentucky. As has been the custom for probably a century, they turned a portion of the conference into a massive prayer meeting primarily for those in need of physical healing. I was unable to travel to Kentucky due to my weakness, but was not forgotten. That night as they prayed, in unison they turned their prayer attention toward me. They called out together for "one touch" upon my body. "One touch" is all I needed from God, and I would be completely restored.

Gary Benedict, the president of our denomination, personally called me after the service that night, blessed me with gracious words of encouragement and told me of their passionate prayers. Looking back, I see this as yet another sweet gift that the body of Christ gave to me.

However, while they prayed I didn't sense anything. In fact, I distinctly remember on that night feeling as low as I had ever felt. I was sick, lonely, irritated, restless, and confused.

*How could so many people cry out to God on my behalf and I not feel any benefit from it? Does prayer work? Is God there?*

Simultaneous to my disappointment, however, I also knew something else. It may be that the Christian church has always struggled with this issue, but it seems that the church in America is ever in search of a formula. We want quick fixes and clear answers. We want certainty. We want control.

I sensed in my spirit, *If God touched me on the night all those people were praying for me, we'd probably mishandle the event and try to turn it into a formula. Across the country the word would spread that if you get enough people together at the same time and they all pray in agreement, then God will heal immediately.*

I don't know for sure that people would have responded to a miracle that way, but I do know that we love formulas. I heard them almost weekly.

Since the doctors hadn't figured out what had nearly killed me or how to fix me, many other people decided to give it a try. It was obvious their efforts arose out of their love and concern for us. All of these people were well-meaning and their ideas had some merit. We were encouraged to:

- Repent of sin
- Break any curse that might have been put on us
- Try a certain supplement
- Go to a certain healing service
- Have more faith
- Take *this* supplement, it's really powerful
- Try this diet
- Take this other supplement, *it's even better*
- Take communion every day for thirty days

Again, all of these things may have been good to do and, at least in some form, we did try them all. For example, while I really couldn't take communion because of my inability to swallow, Joanna and I did our own form of honoring the Lord's Supper every night for a month. It was a sweet time for us, and a daily declaration of our faith.

However, what began to trouble me was the mentality that some Christians seemed to have and I began to be infected with: if we just found the right thing and did it, everything would be better.

At first I was disappointed when one of these efforts didn't seem to "work." I was susceptible to the fallacy many Christians fall into. It seems that as Christians we must be on continual alert that we don't adopt attitudes and behaviors of man-made religions. Across the globe the common practice of countless people is to try to manipulate or appease the spirit world. By giving an offering, saying a chant, wearing an amulet, etc., the human tries to control the spiritual. Biblical Christianity frees us from this kind of behavior, but its subtleties can slip into our theology and practice. We tend to create if/then scenarios: "If I do this, then God will do that."

The God whose ways are higher than our ways and whose thoughts are higher than our thoughts (Isaiah 55:8) can't be minimized in this way. As a friend of mine, Randy Corbin, says, "God reserves the right to be mysterious."

So, while I did what my well-meaning friends suggested I do, I began to believe that God was writing His own story and wasn't going to be manipulated by our human maneuverings. He was up to something, and I had to trust Him. Any sudden answer to prayer or rapid response to our well-intentioned efforts at this point would only have driven me to rely on the method rather than the Master. I don't believe I was ready for a miracle. I know God wasn't, or He would have granted one.

I was called to deeper faith in the midst of uncertainty. I was challenged to trust Him when I could neither see Him nor much evidence of Him. I was being reduced to the most foundational place of trust: would I believe He is good, whether or not I was circumstantially experiencing anything that felt good?

Over and over I declared it during these months, "God is in this and He is good."

Over and over I would be challenged to keep believing my own profession. His goodness wasn't something I could always see or feel.

Some people disputed my "God is in this" statement. They concluded that I was attributing my illness to God. They believed that He would not do such a thing.

I wasn't blaming God or attributing my illness to God. I didn't pretend to know what had hit me. Satanic attack? Some bug from Brazil? Had I worn myself down with my high level of activity? I didn't know and still don't know.

But what I do know is that I can't leave God out of the scenario. My life is in Him and His life is in mine. *In Him we live and move and have our being,* Paul taught in Acts 17:28. He reinforced this teaching in other passages, *I am in Christ* (see Ephesians 1:3-14) and *Christ is in me* (Colossians 1:27).

How could I believe these things to be true but then say that He had nothing to do with this illness? At minimum, He allowed it. I was beginning to suspect that He had even desired it.

God is not the source of evil, but no evil is outside of His jurisdiction. I didn't know exactly what I should think and believe about God's involvement in my situation, but I knew that I couldn't believe that my illness was beyond Him.

No. He was in this—somewhere, somehow—and He can only be good. To believe anything else would have been to fall into ultimate despair.

On more than one occasion, I would adopt the words of the Apostle Peter as my own. Jesus had just preached a controversial message which led to serious conflict (John 6). As large crowds of one-time Christ-followers—now confused and angry—walk away from Him, Jesus looks at His remaining men and says, "You're not going to leave, too, are you?"

I can almost see Peter look around the circle at the other men. They are a discouraged and confused lot. They aren't too pleased with their Messiah at the moment. With a shrug of his shoulders, Peter answers for them all, "Where else shall we turn? You alone have the words of eternal life."

*God, I don't get this. You are confusing the daylights out of me right now. I don't like my life. I can't figure out what you are doing. But with Peter I declare that I have no other place to go! Every other option besides you is a dead end.*

# REASSIGNMENT

Meanwhile, the days kept passing. Another mile marker. Another day I didn't have to live over again.

Joanna and I did our best to celebrate the conclusion of Drew's excellent high school years appropriately. But, it was impossible for my situation not to hang like a cloud over the events. I hated not being able to participate in his senior year to the degree I had with his older brother and sister, I felt very uncomfortable—physically and socially—in my wheelchair during his graduation, and resented not being able to eat at his Graduation Open House.

But this wasn't about me. We tried our best to honor this fine young man appropriately. We were proud of our son. It gave us pleasure to watch him give an outstanding message in his school's baccalaureate service, sing in a final choir concert, and joyfully trounce across the platform to receive his diploma.

Other events were transpiring as well. Life has a way of continuing to move forward—with or without us. My mother turned ninety and I was deeply disappointed to be the only sibling who wasn't able to celebrate with her in person. Joanna's mother became ill and died within a few months. I hated the fact that I couldn't travel with my wife and support her during this emotion-filled time. My friends were running races I once ran, speaking at conferences I once spoke at, and enjoying opportunities I once enjoyed. Life was moving on for everyone else, but it didn't seem like mine was. I seemed stuck. Completely stuck.

In this I was wrong.

One of Satan's best strategies is to lie to us. It could be argued that it is his only strategy, just slightly nuanced from situation to situation. Some of his best lies—that is, his most effective ones—are the ones that contain an element of truth.

A lie that wanted to dominate my life was simply, "You're stuck. You're never getting out of this. Your present situation is your permanent situation."

I had heard it before. It was back again.

Later I could see the fallacy of this. Either God was going to change my situation or change me in the situation. As long as God exists, change is not only possible—change is inevitable. The story isn't over. Another chapter awaits.

But I didn't know this yet. What I did know was that summer was coming, I wasn't showing much improvement and I needed to make a decision.

And, I had plenty of time to think.

*If I had taken a sabbatical, I could have been gone from the church for three months or even six. But for the leader to be gone much longer than that starts to create issues. I'm not able to re-enter my leadership role at the church yet, and am not showing many signs that I will be strong enough anytime soon. No one has said anything to me, but I know that the board has to be wondering what I'm thinking. I have to consider the health of the church, not just my physical health. Eight months have now passed since I last led the team. I guess I need to let it go.*

My voice was still so weak and pronunciation so poor, people often had difficulty understanding me. Most days I required fifteen hours of sleep. I was dependent on a walker and my wife. Even if my mind was returning to full function, nothing else was. I hoped the day would come when I would once again be in full-time ministry, but for this season it seemed to be the path of wisdom for myself and the church: I would step aside.

I met with the church leadership and explained my rationale. They were gracious and kind as always. They generously accepted my request for a reassignment rather than a full resignation. I hoped I could stay connected to the church. I loved the congregation and staff. I wanted to stay involved in ministry in some way and so I gave a few suggestions as to how I might serve the church in a part-time associate role.

I never asked them, but it became obvious that the members of the church board were relieved that I initiated the conversation and they didn't have to. They appeared to me to be eager to move forward. Soon I was standing with my walker before the congregation giving my announcement.

At difficult moments like this, I've often sighed and reminded myself, *there's no easy way to do a hard thing.*

I felt certain about my decision as I explained to the congregation, over the course of five services, that I was stepping down as lead pastor; but my certainty didn't protect me from feeling sad, defeated, and vulnerable. I had always known I'd leave my position someday, but I never imagined it would be in such a broken state.

I easily assured the congregation that they were in good hands— those of wise leaders and God Himself. It was harder for me to believe that my life was in those hands as well.

I was experiencing an internal wrestling match I would privately battle many times in the next year. On the one hand, I should be delighted that the church I had led was solid enough to effectively move forward without me. The major building project was under construction and on target, good leadership was in place, attendance was up, and the spirit of the church was healthy. I should be honored and glad. How churches or organizations function the year after leaders leave or are removed often says as much about the leaders' effectiveness as the time the leaders were there.

Yet, something within me—a petty, carnal me—felt slighted.

*I guess my leadership wasn't that big of a deal after all. I know they appreciated me at one time, but they seem ready to have me gone.*

My head told me one thing while my emotions told me another.

*You've served well./You've been slighted.*
*Get on with life./Hang on to a grudge.*
*They love you./They're glad you are gone.*

My ego was part of the problem. The proud heart, once stranded on the floor next to a garbage can of vomit, had another test coming: a smaller office, a lesser title, a lower wage, and a greatly reduced job description. I wish I could claim to have been above all these challenges, but I wasn't.

Kathy, my ever-faithful assistant at the church, grieved my changes with me. Her every word and expression dripped of her compassion. She solemnly packed up my books from the office suite where we had served side-by-side for seven years, and moved them down the hall and around the corner to a vacant office.

Meanwhile, with summer upon us, our neglected yard was revitalized by numerous volunteers spreading bark, removing a dead tree and planting a dogwood and flowers. Inside, Handyman Jack kept showing up to make another repair or upgrade for us. One lady I barely recognized brought us an exquisite plant adorned with carefully selected scriptures. Two groups from the church, hearing that my legs were too long for our recliner, gathered money for us to buy a chair that fit me perfectly. And, the blog community continued to pour out their verbal support.

If I could just appreciate the body of Christ with all of her expressions of love for us, and not get stuck in the corporate side of the church and my changing position in it, all would be well. I'm not the first nor the last person to struggle with the structure called "the church" at the very moment I was being blessed by the people called "the church."

# TURNING A CORNER

My life at the church wasn't the only thing changing at the time. I wrote a blog entry that described one major change, but I never posted it. Ironically, it was titled *A Subject We Don't Talk About*.

The subject? Depression.

It struck me that we can freely share in a prayer meeting if we've been diagnosed with cancer, but are far less likely to tell the group we're depressed or struggling with other forms of emotional issues.

Depression wasn't a new issue for me. There were three distinct times in my past when I battled with it. Each of these battles lasted a couple months and was overcome without medication. A good exercise routine, taking a few vacation days, getting more sleep, honest communication with a trusted friend, getting out from under unnecessary pressures, better eating habits, going deeper in prayer and the scripture, and other such practical steps became the tools God used for my recovery. It was also essential for me to identify why I had slipped into this dark place. The reasons varied from time to time but all centered on the fact that I wasn't taking proper care of myself.

However, this round of depression had a different feel to it. Months earlier, as I was coming out of my long hospital stay, Dr. Byrkit talked to me repeatedly about taking anti-depressant medication. Knowing all that I had gone through, he believed this to be a wise prescription. He tried to explain to me that certain chemicals in my brain may have been depleted through all that I had endured. I objected. I argued. I declined.

I appreciated his concern, but felt I could handle it as I had in the past. There was no question that I was again battling depression, but I figured that in time I could beat it.

I did okay for a few months. I was struggling, but staying on top. However, as summer arrived I sensed I was fighting a losing battle. My normal strategies were more difficult to maintain and less effective than they had been in the past. I knew I was in trouble when my thoughts started to turn toward self-destructive behavior. I didn't act on these thoughts in any way, but my mind was becoming an increasingly dark battle ground.

With great disappointment that I had reached this point, I talked to Dr. Byrkit about taking him up on his recommendation. There was evident relief in his voice. He prescribed an anti-depressant immediately. He would start me with a mild dose—just one pill. We could increase the dosage if needed, but we'd start small. The pill could be ground up, dissolved in water and poured into my feeding tube. I agreed to submit to his plan.

Dr. Byrkit and Joanna felt hopeful. To me, it felt like total defeat.

*If the joy of the Lord is our strength, why do I need chemical assistance? If I were a stronger person or more spiritual, couldn't I get through this on my own? I always had in the past. Where was God in all of this?*

My reluctant decision to accept the medication came from the following rationale:

- I knew I couldn't keep going as I was. Something had to change. My thoughts were becoming too dark.
- I had previously decided to use every resource available to me in my recovery. Why not try this?
- If my doctor was correct that a chemical had been depleted in my brain, why wouldn't I want to restore it?

I'm not saying that everything the medical community advises is wise. I don't pretend to know who would benefit from doing what I did and who wouldn't. I've heard horror stories of people who end up taking a handful of such medications and have great difficulty ever getting off of them.

But within two months I discovered that I was in a better mental state. This gave me the ability to be more proactive with the practices of self-care, like physical exercise, I'd always found beneficial.

It is my lay opinion that anti-depressant medications helped me regain a state of mind where I became more proactive in doing those things that build long-term mental health. Wrongly used, such medications serve as a cover-up for the true condition and self-neglect. Wrongly used, they mask pain, and give me less reason to begin healthy practices. Properly used, they become a launching pad to better life management.

At the six month mark I was ready to ask my doctor to taper me off, which he did without me experiencing side effects.

*Hmm. Maybe he was right. Think of that. Maybe I did have a chemical that needed to be re-established within me.*

The fact that I turned to an anti-depressant will no doubt come as a disappointment to some, and be a source of encouragement to others. I think it's pretty obvious how this has worked out in my life, but I don't pretend to have a clue what is right for anyone else. I know that this is complex territory, but I promised an "honest look," and didn't feel like I'd be completely honest if I left out this topic.

During the same time period, my doctor began to move away from strong medications like Prednisone, and prescribed an infusion treatment called IVIG. Taken from the plasma of the blood of a thousand donors, this specialized treatment has been known to help rebuild the immune system. Since my immune system evidently attacks itself, this seemed like a good thing to try.

The treatment is slow, four or more hours a day for three days a month, and the results are even slower with little change evident for two weeks. But eventually four things became clear:

- The staff in the Salem Hospital's infusion center is the finest collection of nurses and CNAs ever to be found and,
- The expensive packets of clear liquid were having a good impact on my body. Medically, the IVIG infusions became the most hope-giving treatment I've found for a person in my condition,
- I'm deeply grateful for those who donate blood and plasma,
- And, the captivity of an infusion chair also served as a good place to write. Much of this book was written with an IV in my arm.

Meanwhile, our son, Josiah, came home from college for the summer. Like a pied piper, he drew friends into our house night after night for evenings of worship and prayer. Life, noise, laughter, music, and the slamming of the refrigerator door echoed through our house. Josiah always made sure it was okay with us to fill our home again with his friends. It always was. I wanted our home to be used for such purposes. And selfishly, I wanted to be the recipient of their prayers.

One night, well past my normal bedtime, I reclined in my chair and raised my hands as best I could as twenty twenty-somethings and teenagers surrounded me. They crowded in close around my chair, prayed over me, and then broke into song. Their singing somehow turned into prophesying as—loudly and repeatedly—they declared the words from an old camp chorus:

*Spring up oh Well, within my soul.*
*Spring up oh Well, and make me whole…*

Their young faces exuded joy. Their spirits filled the room with faith. Their song kept echoing in my heart.

I envied their youth. I envied their health. I envied their ability to eat. I envied most their faith.

I wanted to grab onto their joy and make it mine. I wanted to truly rejoice again, and not have every statement of praise arise from a determined act of my will. I wanted to *be joyful* not just choose to give God praise because it was the right thing to do.

I wanted to minister to these young adults, be an example for them, and to give a "word" to them. Instead, they were the ones ministering to me. I had nothing to give. I only hoped I could receive.

# SAME ROAD, DIFFERENT PERSON

"These three remain," Paul taught. "Faith, hope and love" (1 Corinthians 13:13).

Faith and hope were hard to find in my heart during these summer months. Gratefully, love—through God's people—was still very obvious. And according to Paul, "The greatest of these is love."

God felt invisible to me. I couldn't seem to hear His voice, feel His joy, or experience His presence.

I searched through Isaiah until I found a verse I knew was there, but never appreciated as fully as I did now.

"Truly you are a God who hides himself" (Isaiah 45:15).

I don't know what Isaiah was experiencing as he penned those words. I do know they resonated deeply within me.

*God, where are you?*

Meanwhile, He kept finding ways to show up through His body. I wanted GOD to show up, and it's as if He wanted me to understand that He was present...through His people.

Later, a church elder would humbly say to me, "I believe I have a word to give to you: 'Let people minister to you.'"

Oh. That's never been easy. I feel better doing the ministry, rather than being on the receiving end. I would ask myself, *Are we truly prepared to give if we are resistant to receive?*

So, while faith and hope were at an all-time low, love kept showing up on our doorstep. One such loving expression came through a couple in the church who offered us a week at their time-share condo on the Oregon Coast. They had a schedule conflict and couldn't use it, or so they claimed. Would we benefit from it?

Joanna and the boys liked the idea. I was hesitant. To be more accurate: I was afraid.

Most chairs were very painful for me to sit in. Some bathrooms were very difficult for me to use. Other daily issues of life, that I had figured out how to manage in our home, loomed as great unknowns. For a lifetime I had travelled the globe from Saharan desert to Amazon rain forest with free-spirited pleasure. Now, I feared someone's well-equipped condo one hour's drive away. My world had shrunk so rapidly.

Yet, there was one factor greater than my fear: I didn't want to spoil the one chance the family would have to experience a semblance of a vacation this summer. Arrangements were made, the van packed, and on an overcast day in July, Joanna, the boys, and I headed west.

Down the same road to the Oregon Coast that I had started this journey on, we travelled. Virtually nothing had changed, except me.

There's something about specific smells, sounds, or scenes that can stir up emotion. Our memories of certain events—and all the powerful feelings that accompany them—are triggered by the senses. The hour drive I had enjoyed en route to my study break nine months earlier, now felt so vastly different. I rode in the passenger's seat like a victim returning to the scene of the crime.

As we approached the Coast, my body ached from what felt like a very long ride and my apprehensions grew. I wasn't just worried about the logistics. I had to face the reality of my story head on. I was not the same man that I was the last time I travelled this road, and I didn't have a healthy perspective on it yet. I was determined to not spoil the good time awaiting the others, but I was simply hoping to survive. This was not a week to enjoy, but merely endure.

"If it doesn't work for you, we can always come home early," Joanna assured me.

I was grateful for the escape plan, but didn't want to have to use it. So much heaviness had hung over our home for so many months, the family could benefit from a change of location.

I've always admired the way my wife and kids don't need to be entertained. They can find plenty of positive ways to fill their time most any place they find themselves. Days at the condo proved to be no exception: books were read, trails explored, crab caught, naps relished, and relaxation enjoyed. A few gray whales even put on a daily show for us outside our picture window.

I continued my practice of sleeping fifteen hours a day, tried to write something for my blog, and spent many hours staring out the window from a chair that worked for me.

Every day I watched the ocean's waves roll in with all their power and unstop-ability. Each wave had a unique pattern, but all found rest on the same sand and then mysteriously receded back to the depths from which they came. Back and forth. Back and forth. Hour after relentless hour. Every movement utterly unique while being unrelentingly the same.

It was glorious; it was tedious. It was majestic; it was monotonous. It was soothing; it was irritating.

How could the same set of eyes see the same scene and have such a contrasting response?

I watched numbly. Nine months earlier I had been inspired by the view as my mind and fingers raced for thirteen hours a day, writing my dissertation. The contrast of my productivity now was as great as the contrast of my reaction to the waves. For a man who had often measured his success and worth by the amount of work he accomplished in any given day, this was a demoralizing place to be.

I'd confess to the online community in these days that I had a "blog clog." My numbed mind could think of little to say. I tried to stay as positive as I could with the public, but I did admit on one post, "God still seems quite silent—I miss Him."

My emotions toward God ranged from anger to loneliness, from expectancy to utter confusion. Yet, in God's grace, the season of silence was about to end.

By late afternoon each day, I grew restless in the condo. I could only sleep and stare so long. I needed to get outside. The family helped me get into the van and we drove off in attempt to find a few places of interest, two of which quickly became our favorites. One was a paved trail through the sands, tall grasses, and wind-beaten trees of a state park. The boys and Joanna took turns pushing me in the wheelchair for the two-mile hike. I tried not to think too much about what it would have been like to run the trail. It was short, but it would have been fun…last year.

The second destination I immediately appreciated was a pier. Decades earlier, some water-loving city fathers had invested tax dollars to give their citizens a place to throw out a fishing line or crab pot. Others of us enjoyed simply having a level place to feel the wind in our faces and breathe the salty air.

The pier appeared to stretch out for some seventy-five yards. The rough boards of the walkway were solid but irregular—warped and weathered over the decades. A sturdy railing, chest high, guarded the entire length. The pier was wide enough for four people to pass each other. Foot and bicycle traffic were consistent but not congested.

On one of our first times there, I asked the family if they minded if I walked a section of it alone. They could go on ahead or explore other places. I'd follow at my own pace. They could come back and get me in twenty minutes or so. Joanna was hesitant at first. My legs were weak and my balance poor. I hadn't been anywhere without my wheelchair or walker. Was I sure this was a good idea?

I didn't know if it was or not. I just knew that this was the kind of setting I deeply missed. Some of my life's greatest moments of joy and intimacy with God had descended on me in the convergence of physical exercise, solitude, and God's creation. Like a perfect storm, these three elements often collided with gales of life in my spirit.

Inching my way along a boardwalk while being passed by dozens of people hardly qualified as "exercise" and "solitude," but this was the closest encounter I'd had with them in nine months. I'd take what I could get. Besides, the air was good. My face and lungs welcomed it like an old friend.

Clinging to the railing, I shuffled along. I'd stop, breathe as deeply as my weakened lungs would allow, and make my way a little farther down the pier. Like wisps of wind, peace made some passes by my soul.

Suddenly my left foot caught the lip of a board. I stumbled forward, catching the railing with my left hand and arm. I was stuck, leaning forward at about a 70 degree angle. My arm, already too weak to push me upright, weakened further each second as it bore my weight. I knew that if I lifted one leg to attempt to straighten myself up, the other would give way and I'd fall completely. Blood began to stain my sleeve, revealing that I had taken a layer of skin off my forearm in the process.

I gripped the railing, unable to move without falling forward.

*God?*

A middle-aged couple approached from the opposite direction. I caught the man's eye. He immediately read my predicament—a frail man teetering, about to fall on his face—and he gave me the support I needed to stand upright again.

"Thank you," I whispered, embarrassed but grateful. "Thank you."

I wanted to explain. I wanted him to know that the ultra-marathon jacket I was wearing was evidence of the real me. I didn't know this man with a frail body and bloody sleeve any better than he did. I was an athlete and a minister, not this broken stranger needing help!

Yet none of this was said. There was neither opportunity nor strength to say it.

Meanwhile, I was truly grateful for his gracious intervention. I do not know how much longer I could have held myself without falling. He was one more evidence that God would give me what I needed, often at what would seem like the very last moment before I utterly crashed.

My walk was over for this day, but on the next day and every one after that for the rest of the week, I'd ask the family to take me back to the pier, and grant me another chance to have more "exercise" and "solitude" amidst God's creation.

I edged along the railing with more care in the days that followed. I knew that if I fell, my walking privileges would be taken away. I consciously worked on lifting the toes of my left foot and not letting my foot drag. Often, though, I'd simply stand with my chest leaning on the railing and let the wind caress my face.

It was during one of these moments that I sensed I heard God's whisper.

How can a voice be inaudible? I don't know. I just know that in the past I had sensed words landing on my spirit in a way more powerful than audible words passing over eardrums. I "heard" this voice again as I leaned against the railing:

*You've been given a challenge. Rise to it.*

Simple words. Anyone could have said them to me at anytime in this journey, and they would have been equally as accurate...but I would have ignored them. Words processed only by our heads, words that come through the eye or ear gates but only go a few inches farther, don't change us. It is the words that somehow arise within our spirit and then move into our soul and mind that change us.

I had heard the words, accompanied by their reassuring comfort and courage, and I was truly helped. Just as days earlier a passerby had lifted up my sagging body, now a "parakletos" lifted up my sagging spirit.

Forgive me for throwing in a word from the Greek New Testament at this point in the story, but Jesus refers to the Holy Spirit as the "parakletos" in the Gospel of John (see John 14:16; 14:26; 15:26; 16:7). This description of the Holy Spirit reveals that the Spirit is our Helper, our Advocate...the One walking alongside us every step of the way through our journey of life. There is no road or trail or hallway or pier that He has not walked with you.

His presence is often hidden from our awareness, but real nevertheless. In His kindness, as I leaned on the railing and stared out over the water, He broke the months of silence.

Yes, it was true. I *had* been given a challenge. It wasn't easy, but neither was it by accident. He was involved. I wasn't alone. And, I had my part to play—a response was being called out of me.

*Rise to it.*

As silently and mysteriously as the "voice" came, it was gone. But I had heard. I had been helped. I would accept the challenge.

What I gained from that brief encounter with the Holy Spirit on the pier was a new perspective. Nothing circumstantially had changed. But now I had some insight on what was happening. It was simple. It was profound. It was what I needed.

And, in God's kindness, it was coupled with another personal insight. God's whisper wasn't confined to the pier.

We finished our time at the condo and returned home with a glimmer of hope. The family had all benefited from the change of pace and environment that the gift of the condo had provided. And, I think they detected a slight lift in my attitude as well.

# A BETTER VIEW

I'm the kind of person who often thinks in pictures. Some authors call these mental pictures of life "metaphors." I knew from the writing of others and my own personal reflections that these metaphors could either be energizing or debilitating. How I perceive a situation inspires or discourages my spirit.

Through these long months of slow recovery, I was aware of several harsh mental pictures that kept arising within me. Instinctively, I responded to my dramatic change of events by picturing myself as having been hit across the head with a baseball bat. A friend of mine, a brother who otherwise was often very helpful in this journey, kept using another very unhelpful metaphor, "Man, you were just going about your life, when out of nowhere…WHAM! You were run over by a semi-truck! You were clobbered!"

I couldn't argue with him. His description felt accurate…but completely unusable.

Whenever he'd say it, I kept thinking, *No. I don't want to view myself that way.*

Yet, how was I to view my situation? What mental picture was both accurate and uplifting?

I prayed about it on more than one occasion.

*God, you know I think in pictures. You know I don't want to keep seeing all this as a whack across the head or getting run over by a truck.*

*What is accurate? What is really going on here?*

I can't tell you how many times I prayed this or how many weeks passed, but quite uneventfully, as I reclined in my chair at home, an ancient and empowering metaphor came to me. Over the months that followed, I'd come back to the picture time after time.

With growing clarity and with greater detail than I had "seen" the baseball bat or truck, I could "see" hands shaping a pot on a wheel. Wet clay was being carefully molded as it spun. Damp hands held it firmly and skillfully. The pot in the hands already stood a couple feet high. I liked the pot. It had no special elegance to it, but it looked strong, sturdy, functional...nearly complete.

Suddenly, as the wheel and pot continued to spin, the hands pressed firmly down on the clay. In almost an instant, the well-established pot was now reduced to a few inches tall with the thumbs of the hands almost touching the base.

Mysteriously—without comment or explanation of any kind—the Craftsman had decided to start over; not from scratch, not discarding the clay all together, but from an unglamorous lump, He was beginning anew.

Over the weeks I would ponder, *The first pot looked perfectly fine to me. Why did He have to reduce it down?*

Without question, I knew I was the clay and God the Master Potter. The message was clear, personal, and perspective-bringing.

No, I hadn't been beaten nor run over. I was in good hands...artistic hands. The base was still spinning, the work was continuing. I was being re-formed. The Creator Himself was re-shaping my life.

*But I liked my old life just fine! I liked the old pot!*

My guess is that God heard my complaints and just sighed a gracious—"trust-me-I-know-what-I'm-doing"—smile. You can picture it, can't you? It's the smile a sweet grandmother gives—if she's not completely worn out herself—when she knows the children are desperately tired and will feel much better if they go to sleep, even though the kids don't understand why she would be so strict as to enforce a bedtime. It's the I've-done-this-lots-of-times-and-know-it-works "sigh smile."

Summer ended with abruptness. Suddenly our two sons stood at the front entry of our house, laden with backpacks and suitcases. The fall semester of college was beginning—Josiah's senior year and Drew's freshman. We hugged good-bye. A friend drove them to the airport. They were gone. The nest emptied in a moment.

It pained me deeply—it angered me—that I couldn't do for Drew what we'd done for his older siblings. As Anna and then Josiah launched their college years, we turned the events into family vacations and personally handed our kids off to the colleges of their choosing. These are family highlight moments I cherish to this day. For me, the college-hand-off was a rite of passage experience, and was a significant component of my parenting role.

Now, with a prayer, a couple hugs, and the close of the door, they were gone. After twenty four years of the noise, activity, life, and love generated by children among us, our home was quiet. Profoundly quiet. Joanna went into our room and closed the door. I knew she needed to grieve alone for a while. I reclined in my chair and pouted.

In God's kindness, He gave us the will and energy to do more than just grieve and pout over this new era of life. Yes, we would continue to feel the loss of the end of our kid-in-the-house parenting, but I was buoyed by the improved perspective the Lord had given to me. Meanwhile, Joanna kept showing amazing perseverance and gave me great support.

Our activity level slowly began to increase along with our spirits. The monthly IVIG infusions seemed to be helping. Joanna and I were now making almost nightly trips to walk a new path opened by the city. City leadership had transformed an old railroad trestle into a pedestrian bridge, and we took full advantage of it.

I still fought with muscle weakness and pain, never-ending skin rashes, the inability to swallow and the oppressive sense of "just being plain-old sick." However, I had real signs of progress.

I announced to the blog community,

> The biopsy-gone-bad wound is now just two little scabs the size of a fingernail. I think it is time to declare that it is healed! It took seven months, but I had no complications or infections. My only disappointment is that my scar isn't as big as the original wound. But, I do have pictures. It's a guy thing.

Of even greater significance to me is my improved walking. I know that some of you think I'm "off my rocker"—but now I'm officially off my walker! It's been retired—hopefully for good. I've graduated to a cane and it is going well.

Psychologically and physically this is a big win for me. Joanna and I walk Salem's new pedestrian bridge a few times a week and the treadmill keeps me going when we don't get out. I can walk a mile fairly easily now. A friend reminded me that just a few months ago it was a major accomplishment that I walked the fifty feet to our mailbox with my walker, and now I can do the whole bridge and back. Your prayers have not been in vain.

On Friday I get my feeding tube changed. The nurse assures me that this is a "no big deal" routine procedure, but anything that involves invading my stomach leaves me feeling a little unsettled. The first time they put it in at OHSU I was incoherent. This time I'll be a fully awake out-patient. I'll let you know how it goes.

Joanna continues to serve me with strength, patience, and grace. Thanks for continuing to uphold her in prayer as well.

Our love to all of you,

John

# ON THE TUBE AGAIN

Friday came too soon.

"Do they do colonoscopies in this room?" I asked.

"Yeah, they do," my friendly male nurse answered.

I thought it looked all too familiar. Tubes, hoses, machines, and monitors surrounded me as I stretched out on the hospital bed. I remembered the "decorations" too.

*Even though it is a hospital, do they really need to decorate the walls with body part posters?*

Yes, indeed. I had been here before. I should have asked if they offered discounts for frequent users:

*Come back in the next sixty days, and receive 25 percent off the procedure of your choice.*

As my nurse went through some paperwork, I broke the silence, "Do you do this procedure very often?"

I was trying to tactfully approach the subject as to whether he was a veteran at this or not. I had been a live dummy for medical novices before, and wasn't in the mood for that today.

"We do them all the time," he assured me.

Gerry, another kind male nurse, entered the room and discussion ensued for the next ten minutes as to the oddity of my disease and the uniqueness of my current feeding tube—it didn't have the normal identifying markers typical of most tubes. By their comments, I gathered that they had never seen one quite like it before. This was not reassuring.

"It's from OHSU," I said, figuring that would explain everything.

They soon decided on what size tube they would use for replacement, and then informed me that they would need to gown up because sometimes stomach fluid squirted out in the process. I pictured a miniature geyser spouting out of the hole in my abdomen dousing us all. My new friend put on a gown, gloves, and a nifty mask and face shield combination that made him look more like a welder than a nurse.

"Okay," he explained. "You're going to feel me making it tight, and then I'll give it a yank."

"Wait a minute," I objected. "Aren't you going to deflate the balloon?"

Somewhere I had picked up the idea that an inflated balloon device held the tube in my stomach.

"Oh, you don't have that kind," he patiently responded. "You have a button that collapses as I pull it out. I'm told that it hurts, but only for a moment."

Well, he was right on the first half of that sentence anyway.

I reclined in the bed, grabbed the handrails and felt the forewarned tightening. Suddenly, WHOA! I was momentarily lifted off the bed as he ripped the button out of my belly. It hurt alright—an inside the body, I'm glad I don't feel this way every day—kind of hurt.

I leaned forward to see him holding my old feeding tube with a rubber disk about the size of a quarter at the end. His mask and gown were perfectly clean. No geyser. How disappointing. I always thought my gut was kind of wimpy—getting motion sick on fair rides and boats. Here was its big chance to spout off, and it just laid there writhing in pain.

"The bleeding is normal," Gerry assured me as I watched the red pool form in what was now just a hole right under my rib cage.

He then pulled out a bottle of liquid and poured it on the area.

"This will numb it a little bit," he explained.

*Now you give it to me,* I thought but kept my mouth shut.

*I could have used a little of that five minutes ago when Captain Yank was doing his work.*

Like a worm boring into the ground, a new tube was inserted through the hole with only mild discomfort.

"We gave you the balloon kind this time," my nurse announced. "This kind will come out a lot easier when you have to have it replaced again, but they tend to wear out faster, too. If it comes out on its own, get to the hospital right away because the hole starts to heal in twelve hours, and if it heals they have to start all over and go down through your throat."

My kind nurse slowly walked me back to the lobby to meet Joanna who had opted out of watching the procedure—believing she had seen enough of the medical world lately.

I hoped that the next time I found myself back in that room would be a day of celebration. I wanted to eat again. I wanted to eat again very badly. I resented this device that hung hidden under my shirt. I began to think of it as a parasite attached to my body.

But, I tried to cling to the hope that one day I would indeed swallow and have no need of my "parasite."

# NOTHING ANYONE CAN DO

I tried to find humor in my situation any time I could. Laughter helped counter-balance the heavy emotions with which I lived. Sadly, I could not sustain my humorous approach. For every time I laughed about my condition, there were a dozen that I struggled. Here is a sampling of my reactions to what I came to call *A Life I Couldn't Swallow:*

———∞———

I'd rather not even go inside. My family has stopped for a fast food lunch. They need to eat. I understand. The world can't stop just because of me. Little is said between us. What is there to say? I don't eat. I can't eat. I never eat. Today is no different. While they eat together, I take laps around the van. Shuffling my walker around the parking lot, I count as I go. On lap fifteen they return. Somehow the smell of fries lingers on their clothing. I am helped back in the van. Little is said. What is there to say? I don't like this day.

———∞———

Weeks turn into months. A plastic tube is my lifeline. Corn syrup and chemicals in a can are my nutrition and hydration. I grow to detest the product. I read the same can label over and over, day after dreary day: "medical food" it is called—two words that should never be put together. The burps and gas it produces are foreign…alien. I'm repulsive to myself.

The feeding tube is little more than a piece of plastic with a cap on the end—such a simple invention. By it my life has been spared. I should be grateful that the technology has kept me alive. I am not. It hangs from my stomach and drips its last drops of formula onto my pants. It oozes its leakage from the stomach hole and creates a painful crust on my tender skin. It stinks. Literally. A tall dog sniffs my stomach region with eagerness. I fear that she will attempt to bite it, and rip it from my stomach. The feeding tube is my lifeline, but it is not my friend.

———————

Everyone is chosen to "play" except me.

I already know it to be true, but in a glaring way I come to see how food and beverage are so thoroughly interwoven into our culture...and perhaps all cultures. Food and hospitality, food and friendship, food and conversation, food and meetings, food and celebration, beverage and social interaction, water and exercise...all go together.

What are holidays without special food? What's a date with your spouse without food or beverage involved in some way? What are lunch meetings if no one eats? What are sporting events and birthdays and parties and countless other events without the Cokes or cakes?

A dozen times well-meaning people who know my condition ask, "Can I get you something to drink?"

They catch themselves too late. They are embarrassed. It's okay. But it leaves one feeling like he's lined up on the fence, the teams have been chosen and his name was never called. The game will go on as it always does.

He just won't be playing.

———————

It's the church staff Christmas party. It was always an annual highlight. To laugh, sing, joke, and eat with the team that has labored together for the year brought great pleasure. This year will be different, but I try to make the most of it. I volunteer to provide a game, and attempt to read a humorous story. It fails miserably. With my weak voice and pitiful condition, I don't make a good comedian. Then lunch is served. It's beautiful. Catered. Aromatic. I sit at the empty table as the staff rises to fill their plates.

Josh, a young staff member, kindly pulls a chair up next to me and asks a couple thoughtful questions. I'm deeply grateful for his concern and the distraction he provides. He doesn't mention my inability to eat, but he sits by me and occupies my thoughts with other things while silverware clinks against laden plates.

———∞———

The pastoral leadership team has asked if I'd join them for their retreat. As they go inside Subway to grab a quick lunch, I stay outside in the van. I've poured formula down my feeding tube in public before, but have received some upset looks from restaurant customers. I can't say that I blame them. Feeding tubes look like they belong in hospital wards not restaurant booths. I won't make another scene today—especially with the team. My three cans of formula go down quickly. As the sun pours in through the passenger window, I wait. There's nothing they can do. It's just the situation we find ourselves in. I'm not sure I should be here.

———∞———

Another holiday arrives. Holidays and food are best friends. The one only enhances the other. We're in a home. The décor and atmosphere are as festive as the aromas. By now, I've become skilled at what my speech/swallow therapists call "recreational eating"—chewing on food and then spitting it out. The odd practice is cautiously authorized by therapists for some patients who can handle food without letting it slip down their windpipe into their lungs. It prevents the patient's chewing muscles from completely atrophying and gives the patient the sensory pleasure of tasting small amounts of carefully selected food.

The family is gracious enough to allow me to sit at the table and spit into a plastic container. I try to be as inconspicuous as possible. I fear that to some at the table my practice is disgusting, but I accept the offer of the host with gratitude. I cannot swallow, but I can at least taste. I've "eaten" a meal without consuming a calorie.

In time, I slip away from the table to find a quieter place for my formula and feeding tube routine.

———∞———

Publically I make jokes about recreational eating.

"You'd do it too if you hadn't eaten since the Bush administration!"

But privately, I hate it. It is so unsatisfying. I chew almost an entire bag of Doritos, spit them back into a container and dump the remains down the garbage disposal. This is just wrong. I feel like I've developed a new form of eating disorder—it's bulimia's ugly cousin.

———∞∞∞———

It's evening. I sit in my chair surrounded by a day's work and tomorrow's stash. Defiled napkins, paper towels, and spit rags are my handiwork. Hour after relentless hour, my body generates saliva I can do nothing with but eject. I hate the choking feeling I experience every time the saliva slips into my windpipe. Spitting is nonoptional.

I can identify different styles of saliva based on the hydration level of my body. I generate one type of saliva that makes strands that can stretch a yard long. I've made designs with it into the napkins. I can identify different brands of paper towels by their spit absorbency and the chemical residual that some seem to leave on my skin. I am an expert in things I hate.

I'm standing in the produce section of a large grocery store. Joanna needs supplies and I tag along to get out of the house. I encourage her to go ahead of me and I'll meet her at the appointed time. I stand and stare.

The vivid colors of God's incredible creations splash across the canvas before me. The scene looks absolutely beautiful. The gleanings of a hundred gardens and groves are on full display in all their juicy, alive wholesomeness. Tomatoes, peppers—green, red, and yellow—carrots, cucumbers, apples, oranges, watermelon, plums, pears, and peaches are tastefully displayed.

And they mock me.

I can't have any of it. There isn't a single thing in sight that I can eat. There isn't a single thing in the vast store I can eat. There isn't a single thing on the planet I can eat.

And I hate it.

As I stand staring at the produce, a verse I had memorized many years earlier suddenly becomes a prayer—a plea—arising within me,

*God, your Word says that you have given us richly all things to enjoy* (1 Timothy 6:17). *I WANT TO ENJOY THIS! I WANT TO ENJOY THIS NOW! PLEASE LET ME EAT!*

Heaven seems silent.

I slowly walk the store's aisles. I am angry.

———⚬⚬⚬———

A person in our church tells me, "I wish I had a swallowing problem. Then I wouldn't be so tempted by food."

I'm stunned. I just look at her and say nothing. Surely she can't mean what she's just said. To have the opportunity—the ability to eat—is to have the potential of temptation.

But, would we really forgo the ability to eat just to avoid the presence of temptation?

I've been on both sides. Give me the temptation, please.

———⚬⚬⚬———

I feel inhuman. Every person I know eats. I alone do not. I had spent months in a wheelchair, but many people share this section of the church with me. Pain rotates through my body, but I know that many people live with pain—some far worse than mine. I fight depression, but know that millions do as well. Where I feel alone, worse than alone—weird, singled out, isolated, a monstrosity—is in the fact that I do not eat. I live, but do not eat. I feel alone in my world.

Everywhere I look, someone is eating. I watch the pedestrian eat a sandwich as he walks. I watch the driver in the car next to us sip a beverage. My son's friends come to our home, the refrigerator door opening and closing every few moments, and the sound pains me. Even the bird out my window eats.

To be alive is to eat. Never in world history, before the invention of the feeding tube, has anyone lived for a year without eating. This is not human. This is not what it means to be alive. I wonder what I've become.

# SOMETHING BETTER THAN RESENTMENT

Now that I was walking freely with the cane, we graduated to the regular pews at church. However, the months in the wheelchair section had been instructive. Each week I was struck by the contented joy I found among those who sat there. I reflected on the fact that the section with wheelchair-bound people and their caregivers seemed to be perhaps the most cheerful section of the church. Somehow, in spite of their infirmities (some of which were worse than mine), they had a lighter spirit than I did each week. I came to conclude that they had reached a level of acceptance about their condition that I had not reached.

For months, I resisted the idea of accepting my condition because I felt it was fatalistic to do so—that it was giving up on getting better. My attitude was, *I'm not going to accept this because I don't like living this way, and I don't want to be this way indefinitely.*

However, resenting my condition did me no good.

I eventually concluded that a better approach was available. I could accept the present while battling for a better future. I began telling myself, *Accept today. Battle for a better tomorrow.*

Paul taught his assistant Timothy, "Godliness with contentment is great gain" (1 Timothy 6:6).

Contentment, I concluded, was not the same as passivity. I was learning to take the step of faith required to accept my current undesirable situation, while doing what I could to improve upon it. I found no value in resenting the day at hand. God was not honored by my resentment, nor was my healing enhanced by it.

Instead, as I submitted myself under the hand of God for daily life—that is, *chose contentment*—I found a semblance of rest.

From this new place of peace—acceptance—I could pray and fight for a healthier future; I could pound on the door of heaven to heal me and work hard at therapy. I realized that an attitude of acceptance need not lead to passivity or fatalism. Instead, it could be the springboard to a proactive effort and a new source of faith.

I wondered how this approach might be applied by those whose finances had tanked, relationships were rocky, emotions raw, or who struggled with loneliness. Perhaps others could benefit by facing their present situation with acceptance *without* waving the flag of surrender as if there was nothing we could do for an improved tomorrow. There always seems to be one more proactive step we can take, tiny though it may feel.

I believe God strengthens us in this step-by-step kind of journey. I believe He is honored when we lift our head toward heaven and declare:

"This is the day—yes, even this difficult day—that you have made. I may not like it, but I choose to accept it and rejoice in it. And, with your help and by your grace, I will do something today so that my tomorrows will be better."

I didn't live with this attitude every hour of every day. I'm not that strong. My emotional responses and my mental processing of my condition would still swing back into the resentment territory, but my "pendulum" was no longer stuck there. It had found better places as well.

And, as my step-by-step journey continued, I had to accept something else: Not every step attempted necessarily led to success.

# PARKING LOT TOURS

I had to at least give it a try. It's a guy thing and after all, it had been more than ten months since I last had the experience.

I remember that it was a Monday. Joanna and I were out running errands. On the way home, at my request, she pulled the van into the local Latter Days Saints' parking lot. It seemed like the perfect location: plenty of room and not another vehicle in sight. Joanna parked, got out of the van, and took the seat I had occupied for all these months. I made my way into the driver's seat, grabbed the steering wheel and breathed a deep sigh; it had been a long time.

My mind raced back through the last decade of teaching our own children to drive. We would typically start them in a vacant parking lot much like this one so that they could get a feel for the experience without having to deal with real life traffic. Now I was the student driver, needing a traffic-free environment.

I noticed Joanna out of the corner of my eye. She seemed hopeful. It was no secret that she would be delighted the day she no longer had to be my chauffeur. Driving has never been her love.

She also seemed apprehensive. Perhaps nearly a decade of teaching teens to drive still had her a little jittery. Or, maybe it was because her cane-walking, tube-feeding, disease-inflicted, physically-impaired husband now had her life in his hands.

Nah, couldn't be. I smiled at her and prepared to head off.

My first indication that this may not go real well was when I couldn't lift my right leg high enough to step on the brake. I had to release my hold of the steering wheel and lift my leg with both hands to get my foot onto the brake. This was not a good sign. With some effort I got the van into gear and backed up. We were on our way.

Using the same hand maneuver I got my foot onto the gas pedal and we headed off at a bold seven miles per hour. Even at that speed the corner came up suddenly, and I turned as hard and fast as my arm, shoulder, and chest muscles would allow.

Wow! Who knew it took so much strength to turn a steering wheel? An involuntary sound emitted from Joanna's throat...some might be tempted to call it a scream. Hope was fading and apprehension was rising...as was the blood pressure.

Next, we headed down the straightaway—a little faster now—perhaps a death-defying ten miles per hour. Straightaways are good. Straightaways are happy. Straightaways require little effort. All too soon, however, another corner was upon us. It was upon us fast. This time I tried the lift-the-leg-onto-the-brake-with-the-hands procedure but had to rapidly get my hands back onto the steering wheel in an effort to make the corner. My muscles screamed. Joanna, with great self-control, did not...but I think she might have cheated and closed her eyes.

Ha! We made it without hitting the curb. It was ugly. I would have taken out any oncoming traffic. But, I was on the straightaway again.

Now it was time to practice parking. I didn't admit it to Joanna, but I missed the spot I was aiming for by three stalls. I angled us in and was taken by surprise by how long it took me to get my leg hand-lifted to the brake. We came to a jerking stop right before driving up onto the curb. I'll admit that an involuntary sound emitted from my throat this time. We won't call it a scream. Real men don't scream, right?

*That was close!*

I imagined how embarrassing it would have been to go to the church and confess that I was the one who defiled their brand new lawn, "Hi, Elder Jones. I'm a pastor here in town and I just ripped up your new sod. Welcome to the neighborhood."

One would think that now that we had found a safe resting place, I would have called it quits. No. For some reason I felt the need to complete an entire circle of the parking lot. Even I marvel myself sometimes.

When I finally completed our little tour, I was exhausted. For the first time Joanna took her eyes off the road. She looked a little white. She didn't object when I suggested that one lap was enough and that I be done for the day.

"Well," I said, back where I belonged in the passenger's seat. "I guess I'm not road ready yet."

Sometimes a guy just has to state the obvious. She agreed in a way that acknowledged the truth without belittling me in the process. I noticed that she seemed more content to be my chauffeur in the days that followed.

I wasn't really surprised that I had failed. I was determined at some point that I'd try again. In the meantime, I'd have to keep working on the physical therapy program and be content to be driven rather than to drive.

My physical therapist was not pleased when she heard of my efforts to get back behind the steering wheel.

"He thinks he's going to be able to drive again!" she told a home health care nurse incredulously.

She knew my muscles were in no condition to do so, and didn't have any reason to believe that my condition was going to improve to the point that I ever could.

I didn't know if I'd ever drive, eat, run, or do the things I once loved doing. The medical professionals around me didn't seem to know either. Only God knew, and although I was coming out of the "dark night of the soul," He remained silent about some of my greater questions.

*What is this all about? Will I ever feel good again? Will I ever eat food again? How is He going to use this long trial?*

But in spite of my unanswered questions, flickers of hope—like fireflies on a summer's night, tiny and intermittent though they be—began to arise in my soul.

Jeff, an elder and friend from church, visited our home each month. Our conversations helped take my thoughts places they couldn't quite reach on their own. I remember telling him one day, "If God heals me of this, I'll be the most blessed man I know to have had this experience. If He doesn't, I don't know what to say about all this; but if He does heal, I'll consider this whole ugly journey a true gift."

# ONE YEAR DOWN

*I think I'm close to Mile 365.*

On many nights, I continued to picture the passing of another mile marker. Another day done. Another "mile" run.

Joanna and I both had a sense of accomplishment when we reached the one year point of our trial. We tried our best to keep too much "severe" from dominating our opportunity to "per-severe." So much had changed in a year's time; so much loss. Attempts at humor had been one survival strategy along the long road. Clinging to each other had been another. The metaphor of the potter re-shaping my lump of clay continued to be of great significance to me.

As our journey started into its second year, I found another picture helpful: the road trip. It occurred to me that sometimes we have to take the long view. Watching the minute hand on the clock is too discouraging. We're helped by switching our gaze to the calendar instead.

From my earliest childhood memories, the Stumbo clan has always been willing to conquer long distances to celebrate a holiday or experience a vacation or preach about Jesus. This need for long-distance travel was accentuated by the fact that we lived for many years in North Dakota and Montana where trips are measured, not by minutes, but by hours and days. Some of my best memories with my parents are nestled in a loaded vehicle on a lonely highway somewhere between Sioux Falls and San Diego.

Decades later, as a father myself, some of my best memories are of another car-full, this time with my wife and three children, travelling through picturesque places such as Kellogg, Idaho, and Gettysburg, Pennsylvania. I love road trips.

Through the years I learned that there is one essential item you absolutely must bring with you for a successful road trip. Sunflower seeds, chocolate, water bottles filled with ice, sunglasses, SunChips, baby carrots, good music, audio books, napkins, a novel, a small blanket, and your favorite pillow are all highly recommended, but you can forget one of them and still have a great trip...if you pack the one essential: *a long distance mindset.*

Few of us come by this mindset naturally. This is partially because we rarely spend more than an hour at a time in a car. Maybe if the traffic is really bad we'll have a little longer commute to work or trip to the airport, but for most of us our time in the car can be measured by the minute hand. However, for a true road trip, we're better off if we forget the watch and pull out the calendar:

*By Tuesday we should be in Albuquerque, and if all goes well, we'll watch the sunset with our toes in the Pacific Ocean on Wednesday... Thursday at the latest.*

Road trips: Think calendar not clock.

Without the essential long distance mindset, we travel restlessly. We never settle in and simply enjoy the ride for the ride, the view for the view, the experience for the experience itself. Without a long distance mindset the road seems like a burden to bear or an obstacle to be conquered. If our children in the back seat don't have this mindset we will be forever hearing the nagging question, "Are we there yet?"

But when we can settle in and enjoy the journey for what it is—not an obstacle to be conquered but an adventure to be explored—the miles become our friends, the road our soul-mate.

Reflecting on this metaphor, I wrote to the blog community,

> Such is the attitude I am trying to take with my illness. Such is the attitude I would encourage anyone in chronic pain to try to find: the attitude of the road master, the cross-country mindset. For those living with pain, marking life by the minute or hour—as relentless as the white lines on the highway—becomes oppressive. Better is the person who can take the long term view. We're on a long road.

Throw your watch in the glove box and pull out your pocket calendar. The journey is going to be a lengthy one, and that's okay. Memories will be made, experiences shared, sights seen, and character built unlike any short ride can provide. Throw on some tunes, pop in a few sunflower seeds, set the cruise control, and notice scenery you've never really paid attention to before. You have a lot of miles to cover. Settle in.

*Are we there yet?*

No, and we probably won't be for quite some time. But that's okay. Rumor has it our destination is well worth the trip.

I found the road trip metaphor especially helpful because people often asked me if I was getting better every day. The honest answer was "no." Some days and weeks brought definite setbacks. However, when I took the long term view, I knew I was making progress.

I now only needed eleven hours of sleep a day, made my way around our house without the cane, and felt the inspiration to resume working on my long-neglected doctoral dissertation. I celebrated that I had moved from the one-pound up to the five-pound dumbbell for my workouts, and that zip-lock bags were no longer prison bars. Water bottles were still impenetrable, but since I couldn't swallow, I rarely found reason to try.

Seeing my improvement, people often tried to encourage me with comments such as, "Every day is a gift from God!" and "Isn't it good just to be alive?"

I admired people who lived with such an attitude, but didn't always share it. And, I knew one simple reason why: I still hadn't fully accepted the fact that God had left me on earth and not taken me to heaven when I was—from a human standpoint—so close to being there.

It's a strange thing to be a Christ-follower, completely convinced that heaven awaits our departure from earth. I found that it is possible for this longing for home—in and of itself a beautiful thing—to become a deficit. I often found myself saying that the "every day is a gift" sentiment was overrated. I would have chosen to race on streets of gold rather than limp across my concrete driveway. I would have rather chosen to eat at heaven's banquet table than pour another can of "medical food" down my tube.

# CONFIRMING THE OBVIOUS

I knew I couldn't swallow; I hadn't for an entire year, so it seemed unnecessary. Yet, the medical professionals around me suggested that I should return to the Salem Hospital for twenty minutes and have the specialists take another look at my swallow function via video x-ray.

Mike was there again to greet us. Mike had been my original speech therapist a year earlier when I was hospitalized, and had given me my first swallow test. I was glad to be under Mike's care again, even if it was just for a few minutes. He has a warm spirit and sympathetic nature. And, he remembered us. It's nice to be remembered.

The nurse seat-belted me into the chair making some comment about keeping the lawyers happy. The medical staff put on their protective vests, and I was seated between an x-ray camera and a monitor. Before me were Dixie cups of barium in different thicknesses. On the very long list of medical procedures a person might have to endure, the Modified Barium Swallow has to be among the simplest and least painful. While other procedures require probing and poking and other punishments, the swallow test simply consists of being spoon-fed minty substances that show up very clearly under x-ray.

As I tried to swallow the first liquid, the monitor revealed all. With incredible clarity, I watched my tongue push the liquid out of my mouth and into my throat. My tongue activated the initial phase of the swallow, but that's where the process stopped. All the muscles and movements required to activate the epiglottis and open the esophagus didn't func-

---

tion at all. The spoonful sat unwelcomed. I was quickly instructed to spit everything out into a cup before it found its way into my windpipe.

We tried again a few times with various viscosities and with my head in different positions, but the results didn't improve. Mike didn't have to say anything. The monitor said it all. I had failed again with flying colors...well, at least in x-ray gray.

I can't say I was really disappointed, because I could already feel what was going on inside my throat: nothing. Joanna came to the procedure with higher hopes, so it was harder for her to watch. She couldn't hold back the tears. It felt to her like we were hitting bottom all over again.

But for me, it merely confirmed that I was interpreting my condition correctly. Whether it was barium, mashed potatoes, ice cream, or my own saliva, this is the result I had been getting for the whole year. Now we watched it life-size on video.

The nurse removed my seatbelt and I told her that if the hospital ever fired her, she could get a job operating a ride at Disneyland. It was obvious that she didn't see much humor in my comment. Humor is risky business.

Mike confirmed that I should cautiously continue my efforts at "recreational eating." He instructed me to keep working on the tongue/swallow exercises that all the therapists had me doing through the months, but I could sense he wasn't certain they would ultimately be of great help. With that "I'm sorry" look in his eye, we parted ways.

The months were passing with no hope that I'd begin swallowing, yet I tried to cling to the messages I had received:

*You've been given a challenge, John. Rise to it. His hands are still on you. The clay is spinning. The Artist is not done yet.*

# GIFTS OF FAITH

Although I was having a difficult time seeing each day as a gift and couldn't eat, I didn't want to be the Scrooge of our family Christmas. Our three children and son-in-law made travel plans to spend the holiday with us. It promised to be a happier Christmas than the previous year which was spent in the hospital.

I've never been the easiest guy to buy presents for. I don't really have any collections, my interests are perhaps eccentric, I'm not one that gets into the latest "gadgets" and I already own enough ties. Every Christmas my wife kindly tries to draw a gift list out of me, and every year I only come up with a few suggestions, some of which—such as socks—fail to make the gift-giver feel much like Santa.

My illness further complicated this dilemma for my family. My already small list had been reduced to almost nothing. Without the ability to do so many of the things I loved to do—run, fish, bike, play tennis, eat… just to name a few—my hobby list sat at an all-time low.

My stubbornness also reduced the length of the list. I was adamant that I did not want the family to buy me new clothes that fit my 140-pound frame. I didn't want to remain this scrawny for the rest of my life, so why should they waste money on clothes I wouldn't wear very long?

Yet, my family, loving people that they are, wanted to give me gifts anyway. Finally, the problem was solved as they decided to give me "gifts of faith"—gifts I couldn't use immediately, but Lord willing, I would eventually.

When Christmas day arrived, I was pleased to unwrap a few fishing lures for the day when I could handle a rod and reel again. Most notably, I received gift cards for some eating establishments I missed—Red Lobster, Olive Garden, Jamba Juice, Cold Stone, Great Harvest Bread, and Baja Fresh.

I checked to make sure none of the cards had expiration dates. I had no human evidence of any improvement in my swallow—having been passed off to my fourth and then fifth speech/swallow therapist. Yet, I continued to look forward to the day when this part of life would be restored to me.

As the New Year came, the cards were merely pieces of plastic waiting in my drawer. We continued to pray that the day would come when they would become much more: pleasant outings, delightful tastes, and fine memories.

I appreciated the spirit behind the gifts, "We believe that you'll eat normally again, Dad." "You're going to swallow again, Honey."

This is what I heard with each card. This itself was a gift...the gift of faith. I just hoped my healing would happen on earth. I doubt they take gift cards in heaven.

On the days when my own faith was hard to find, I reminded myself via my blog/journal,

> Sometimes we can believe for ourselves. Other times it helps to have others believe for us.
>
> Our faith can waver. Our "faith meter" can look like a Minnesota thermometer in January. Then someone comes along who has the faith to believe for us, and the warming breeze begins to thaw our hearts.
>
> If you don't have the faith to see your way through your current crises, hang around people who do. Some of these people can be found in books—read the biography of a saint such as Hudson Taylor or countless others who have walked the road before us.
>
> Others of you are in a place where you can come alongside and believe for someone else who is faltering in faith right now. Don't be shy in expressing your God-confidence when theirs is wearing thin. Don't be obnoxious about it, but buoy them up with your

belief that God is in this trial and He is good. This is a significant ministry. Don't underestimate it.

The gift cards sit in my drawer, but when I see them they are a statement to me: someone believes that a better day is coming. Maybe I can keep believing for another day as well.

Believing with you that God's goodness will be revealed in your trial,

John

The restaurants would have to wait. Meanwhile, more cases of formula continued to be shipped to our door.

I complained about my daily diet to the blog community,

> The ingredients of my formula are: water, corn syrup, canola oil and a whole paragraph of four syllable words with way too many "ates" and "ides" such as "alpha tocopheryl gluconate" and "pyridoxine hydrochloride." Mmm, sounds appetizing, doesn't it? Dinner's on me tonight. I've got plenty to share! One can or two? I impose a strict three can limit. Now I know some well-trained and well-meaning medical person will tell me that these things are all fine and good for my body, but when I look at a food label I'm usually looking for one syllable words like "rice" or "beef." The only four syllable ingredients I'm looking for are ones like "choc-o-late chip."

I was over a year into this meal plan and still hadn't gained back even a pound that I lost. My swallow function still showed no signs of progress. I was slow to accept it, but finally became comfortable with the medical term for my condition: dysphasia.

Again, at an effort to find an excuse to laugh, I explained,

> The word "dysphasia" comes from two Greek words, which when interpreted mean, "Bummer, Dude!"

> No, actually they mean "difficulty" and "to eat." To move food from the mouth to the stomach requires dozens of muscles and nerves to work in a synchronized manner. A few bones even get in on the act. (Who knew I had a hyoid bone?) So, swallowing is no simple task. Next time you take a drink of water, just know that there's a whole lot more going on than you ever imagined.

"I'm sorry about the source of that sigh," Joanna compassionately commented one day. "It's food related, isn't it?"

I had unintentionally exhaled loudly as I walked through the kitchen and smelled the hot chocolate's sweet aroma.

Long term illness brings unique challenges. Pain has a way of eroding the spirit. Dysphasia isolates relationships. The soul is called into battle every bit as much as the body. I had been given new perspectives, but I had to keep fighting.

# DEFINING THE MOMENTS

By February I felt like I was entering a new phase in my recovery, but I didn't quite know how to classify it. I tried to pierce the fog of confusion about my own journey in hopes that not only would I be helped by some clarity, but others would as well.

I knew I had to be cautious, though. The human story is so unique to each individual.

"I'm telling you your story, not hers," Aslan explains to the child in *The Horse and His Boy.* "No one is told any story but their own."

At one level, comparison of our stories is harmful. Questions such as, "Why did God do that for you and not me?" launch us on the wrong pursuit. Like the traveler holding the map upside down, such questions fail to guide us to where we need to be.

Yet, on a different plane, I've been amazed at the parallels our stories share. I assumed that my experience would be of interest, and perhaps even of some help, to those experiencing physical crises, but I eventually discovered that many others could relate their stories as well. People who had experienced the loss of a spouse (through divorce or death), a child (through death or rebellion), the loss of income (through unemployment or the declining economy) and other trials felt a kinship with my experiences.

As I reflected on the first sixteen months of my experience, like a man groping his way through the fog, I began to be able to summarize my experience one step—or phase—at a time.

**Phase One** of my journey, I concluded, could be called "Shock and Awe." I neither could believe nor barely comprehend what was happening to me. I was a healthy guy with healthy habits blessed with healthy genes. How could I spend my forty-eighth birthday on my deathbed?

Often the initial news of a tragedy leaves us so stunned we have no means of processing all that is happening. Too much is coming upon us all at once. Our minds, senses, and emotions are overwhelmed. A scoop, or even a whole truckload, of denial often accompanies this phase.

**Phase Two** started while I was still in the hospital. I call it "Survival 101." It looked like I was going to live, but I had a long way to go if I was going to have the quality of life I once enjoyed. Unable to talk, unable to walk, unable to eat, unable to do virtually anything for myself, I had to accept my dependence on others while striving to regain my strength and abilities. It was an emotionally and physically demanding phase.

This is the phase when the harsh reality of our crisis begins to become "real" to us. We wake up in the morning to face the hard facts: we didn't merely dream this and we're not going to "wake up" from it. We may have no idea of all the implications, but we begin to understand that we have a future we never anticipated. Dread and fear—caped and cloaked—linger in the shadows of our soul, whispering their dark messages to us.

**Phase Three** started in rehab. I call it "The Trajectory of Hope." I felt myself improving almost daily. I was able to read again, walk with a walker, and speak with increasing strength. I participated in the Groundbreaking Ceremony for our new building with great encouragement. I was back with people I loved and had good reason to hope that my health would continue to progress steadily.

I don't know what percentage of people experience this phase of early hope, but some do. We have sufficient reason to believe—or are optimistic enough by nature to simply declare—that we're going to beat this. We were down, but we're coming back! The tornado took down the young couple's home, but the husband holds the weeping wife promising, "We're going to make it, Babe. We're going to be fine."

On rare occasions, this "trajectory of hope" rolls right on upward until the crisis has passed. Often, however, another phase awaits.

**Phase Four** arrived like a weather front. I dub it "Faltering Hope." It resembled what the ancients referred to as "the dark night of the soul."

For months my physical progress stalled and at times worsened. My "every day I'm getting a little stronger" motivation turned to "maybe I'll always be this way; maybe I'll never eat again; maybe I'll never lead again" frustration.

My world had changed, but all the changes seemed like losses. The world around me was moving forward, but I was stuck in an ugly place.

Anger, resentment, and bitterness all take their swipes at our souls during this phase. We're susceptible to ugly behaviors such as taking revenge, holding a grudge, and slandering people with our uncontrolled words. Or, we take our anger inward and become moody, sullen, and depressed.

God—if we're willing to admit it—probably leads our list of those with whom we are angry. He seems uninvolved at the very moment it feels like we need Him the most. He seems silent now when we so desperately need Him to speak. The only thing the human race struggles with more profoundly than God's Word is God's silence. Our faith, of greater value than gold, is being tested by fire (1 Peter 1:6-7). This season, it seems, can last a long time.

**Phase Five** slipped in with the stealth of spring after a long winter. Let's name it "Hope Springs Anew." Nah, that sounds like a Christian romance novel. This was no romance.

I take that back. It is a romance—between God and us—but it doesn't read the way we might expect.

Let me try again. I'd call Phase Five "Four Wheel Drive Faith." That's better. Somewhere in the muck, I found a little traction. My spinning wheels finally hit something solid, and I began to inch out of the crud. It was very slow, and no one single factor seemed to thrust me ahead. It was a combination of factors that inched me forward.

Medically, I explored new options. Nutritionally, after fifteen months on the formula, I experimented with homemade concoctions for my feeding tube diet. Spiritually, empowered by better metaphors, I prayed and studied with new zeal and consistency. Physically, I pushed my therapy harder to recapture some of my past strength. Relationally, Joanna and I kept leaning in to each other, having frank and frequent conversations. Meanwhile, faithful friends continued to pray for me. I knocked on every door that looked like it might have potential. I did what I could. All of these factors converged to gradually lead me to a better place.

Yet, I did all of this without any assurance of where it would lead. Perhaps I should expand my title of Phase Five to be "Four Wheeling in the Dark."

In "The Trajectory of Hope" phase, I had a sense of direction. I was moving upward, which to me meant that I was returning to the place I had been before. I would come back. This crisis wouldn't defeat me. With the help of God and God's people, I'd get back on the road and return to my former life.

However, now in Phase Five, I realized I was off road without a sense of direction. There was no returning to my former life. The crisis had "defeated" me in a sense...not in a final way, but in a life-changing way. There was no returning to the place I had been before, for I was no longer the man I once was.

This is one of the difficulties of surviving a "fire." You emerge from the embers a different person. Others around you have been touched by your trial, but not changed by it to the same degree you have been. When you try to re-enter—when you attempt to resume the place you once held in the world—you may find it more difficult than you'd expect. Relationships, conversations, positions, roles...so many aspects of life feel differently than they once did.

In this four-wheeling phase, I was making a "comeback" of sorts, but it felt like I had to blaze my own trail. Like Abraham when God called him to leave his homeland, I kept moving forward, but had no map. The trail wasn't marked. No signs pointed the way.

I told myself, *Keep one foot moving in front of the other, even though you have no idea where the trail leads. Keep moving. Keep moving.*

I wondered, *Will I ever swallow again on this planet? Will I ever join my daughter and run again with these legs? Will I ever play a competitive set of tennis again with my boys? Will I ever lead a ministry again? Will I ever be free to do all that is in my heart to do? I pray that I will, but I don't know His plan.*

In the midst of this season of questioning, I was given the opportunity to preach again at our church. My text, from the life of Jeremiah, caused me to ask the congregation an application question, "Will we keep doing what is right, even when we don't get the results we expect?"

The question was a very personal one for me as well.

*Would I do what was right, even if I never got any healthier? Would I still trust Him, even if I never swallowed again? Would I keep taking steps of faith and obedience even if I never saw more than one step ahead?*

My hope had no specificity. I hung on to Christ as I think I had always tried to do. But I was accustomed to clinging to "Christ *and* a hope of a better tomorrow." Now it became "Christ...and I don't have a clue about tomorrow."

This is why I've settled on calling this phase, "Four Wheeling in the Dark." I was moving forward, but with extremely limited visibility. Some days it felt like an adventure. Other days it felt like madness.

In Phase Five our newly refined faith is being tested again. We're off-roading, but at least we're not stuck. We're on dangerous terrain, but we're not traveling it alone.

Meanwhile, the continued kindness of God's people served as an oasis and gradually the scriptures were coming to life again. Perhaps the sandpaper's work was complete.

Fresh breezes of encouragement returned. The drought was ending. Reading each day through the Old Testament—a few chapters of history, a Psalm, and a chapter or two from the prophets—along with the writings of the church fathers became surprisingly enjoyable. My devotional time became my best hour of the day. My spirit was being renewed.

It was during this time that I wrote out a prayer that summarized some of my devotional reflections. I called it *A Prayer Inspired by Some Friends:*

Kind Father,

I have been enjoying the privilege of reading of the saints of old. I find your servants in the most interesting places.

What were your finest representatives in Babylon doing in a furnace? Walking around in the flames with you! My furnace is not as hot as theirs, but could I come through this "fire" without even the smell of smoke, unbound and completely whole?

How is it that in reward for decades of faithful ministry, Jeremiah is thrown into a muddy cistern? Thank you for the friends who, like Ebed the Ethiopian, have come to my defense and rescued me from the muck I've found myself in from time to time.

Daniel could have avoided spending the night with the lions. All he would have had to do was close his window! Surely you would have heard his prayers just as well if he prayed privately. But Daniel would be who he had always been and would do what he had always done—despite a death threat. And you were there with him even in the den. Did he get to use one of those lions for a pillow? I want to be like him and do what is right, even if it might lead to negative consequences for me. I can trust you with the outcome, can't I?

I find Job, a righteous man, sitting in ashes while scraping his festering boils with a broken piece of pottery. Do you always treat your friends this way, Lord? I know the answer. It's no. You treat each of us uniquely. I thank you for that. But, I also thank you for the example of a man whose life has fallen apart, but whose faith digs in deeper. "Though he slay me, yet will I trust him," Job declares—teeth gritted or utterly humbled? I want that same resolve.

And then, the unimaginable happens. We find your Son—your only Son—agonizing on a Roman cross. I am to bear mine as well, you have said. I will do so, but only for today. Thank you that this is all you ask me of. I need not attempt to take up tomorrow's cross. Today's cross is my only assignment.

God of Shadrach, Meshach, Abednego, and Daniel; God of Jeremiah, Job, and Jesus; God of fires, dens, pits, ashes, and crosses; God of ages past and God of today, I praise you that the very same Spirit that enabled the saints of old to endure and even thrive in hard places resides in me as well. It was by your Spirit that they endured, persevered, preached, lived, and died. It was by your Spirit that they completed the task you assigned for them. It is by that same Spirit that I may do so as well. This gives me hope. This gives me courage.

Whatever my fire or pit, den or cross, I believe you will grant me what I need to serve you from that place today.

And I know that, in your kindness, not every day is a pit or den.

You bring us to some very pleasant places as well. Thank you. May I be no less ready to serve you from the palace as I am in the dungeon.

You are good and can only be good,

Amen

# TAKING THERAPY TO NEW LEVELS

As my spirit and strength continued to improve, my desire to drive again grew. To calm Joanna's fears, I took a test provided by an occupational therapist to validate that I was road ready. To her surprise and delight, I passed. I returned to the driver's seat cautiously, but safely. Joanna and I both were relieved to have me behind the wheel.

Others weren't so sure. One girl, when she heard that I was driving again, asked her mother, "He still can't swallow! Should he be allowed to drive?"

Meanwhile, I celebrated other milestones of my recovery. They may not sound like major accomplishments, but for me they were morale boosts as well as evidences of physical improvement.

I put on my own socks for the first time in sixteen months. Every other pair I'd worn during that era had been put on by a caregiver, usually Joanna. It took a little "finagling," and a couple of grunts, but eventually I got those stubborn rascals on my feet. Happy day!

Then, while doing some neck exercises assigned by my speech/swallow therapist, I suddenly was able to do my first sit-up. It wasn't pretty. I couldn't do more than one or two. An onlooker might be tempted to call it more of a "rock up" than a "sit up," but, progress is progress even if it wouldn't win a contest.

My freedom to drive and gradual steps toward independence allowed Joanna to go back to work with the school district while I was able to work at the church a little more than half-time. Things were slowly returning to normal. But it was definitely a new normal with a greatly altered perspective on life.

Months earlier, I graduated from physical therapy in my home. I was deemed strong enough to get out and enter the broader world and work of therapists. Home therapists are great and provide a wonderful service, but it was time to venture on to new territory.

The new physical therapy facility was equipped with an underwater treadmill. I was immediately impressed. The water of the small pool soothed my muscles and was usually the perfect temperature for a work-out. Two cameras displayed my stride on a TV monitor. Submerged handrails provided a good measure of safety. Large windows welcomed plenty of light into the room. Mike, my new therapist, explained that the buoyancy provided by water therapy allowed me to more safely rebuild my strength than the jarring nature of many land based exercises.

At first Mike set the treadmill speed at two miles per hour and had me do a ten minute routine. With his trusty wristwatch placed on the ledge beside my spit rag, he instructed me to rotate every two minutes. First, face straight ahead in a normal walk. Next, turn 90 degrees and walk sideways for two minutes. Then, turn and walk backward. And then, another 90 degree turn and walk sideways again. Finally, I rotated back to face the front for two more minutes and I had completed a nice ten minute rotation—working front, back and each side of my lower body. To give my legs a break, he showed me two core and upper body exercises to do in the water and then I returned for another ten minute rotation on the treadmill. Three sets of this and forty-five minutes later, I felt like I had received a genuine workout.

To this regime he gradually increased my speed and added a few other exercises as well. I grew to admire the way Mike, a tri-athlete himself, seemed to know how much he could push me each week. I also appreciated his words of hope.

One day, as my brother-in-law and sister observed my underwater treadmill routine, I didn't have as much strength as in previous workouts. Mike read my discouragement and announced, "There's only one of us in this room that is going to be younger and healthier next year than they are today. You."

I had aged forty years in four weeks during my illness. Mike believed that this aging could and would be reversed. He inspired me to keep giving my workout whatever I had to give.

One day, weeks into our therapy sessions, Mike announced that I was ready for the jets.

*Jets?*

I knew there were submerged circles in the front of the pool, but I had never been curious about what they might be. Mike explained that they were primarily for swimming resistance so that a swimmer could use the pool for individual training. He further explained that he'd start me out at about 20 percent resistance. My competitive spirit was disappointed by the small number.

*Twenty percent! That doesn't sound like much!*

However, I had no time to ponder or complain.

**Whoosh!**

My underwater treadmill now had the added feature of a current flowing against me. My workout was definitely being taken to the next level. My weak legs struggled to march forward against the current.

*It's a good thing he chose 20 percent. If he turned those things all the way up, they would have blown me right off the treadmill all the way to the back of the pool! Once again, Mike seems to know what he's doing.*

Twice a week, I was back in the pool again and feeling the benefit. I loved the sense of progress. Within a few weeks, Mike had me working out at 40 percent resistance and at 2.5 miles per hour.

However, one day Mike was gone. His assistant welcomed me, and said he had the jets set at my normal 40 percent. I was experienced enough at this time that the therapists felt free to leave the room and allow me to monitor my own workout. As he left to assist other clients, I pushed the appropriate buttons to start up the treadmill and the jets.

WHOOSH! The pool had somehow switched from a solid stream to a raging river!

*March, boy, march! You'll be down current in some backwater eddy if you don't keep your head up and feet moving.*

I survived the two minutes of forward movement and turned sideways fighting the current for all I was worth. I looked down at my feeding tube which usually floated lazily at my side. It was now bouncing along the top of the water like an inner tube being pulled by a boat at high speed.

Not a second too soon, it was time to turn again and walk backward. Whoa! Suddenly my swimming trunks were down to, well, you don't need to know where they were down to. I just know that running backward with one hand hanging on to my trunks, while my feeding tube appears to be in a ski race, as a jet stream threatens to blast me into the back wall was too much. I grabbed the hand rails, jumped off the treadmill, turned off the jets and pulled up my trunks.

When my substitute therapist returned and I told him that the jets were stronger this time, he claimed, "It's not an exact science."

Whether jet settings are an "exact science" or not, I never found out. But I did discover that healing is not.

As I've said, everyone's story is their own. Comparison is dangerous. But in my story, the lines have been blurred between the healing that has come to my body via physical therapy, medical assistance, and divine intervention.

I know without a doubt that I would not have recovered to the degree I have had I not been willing to do the hard work and receive the good assistance of physical therapy. To this day, I work muscles that long to pull into the fetal position and remain there. With pain and effort, I stretch and exercise.

Simultaneously, I know that I have benefited as well from the medical community. Some of their efforts were misdirected and unhelpful, but others such as thyroid medication, blood transfusions, and the IVIG treatments have made a marked difference.

However there are elements of this story to which I can only give God the credit. It is my deep conviction that I should continue to ask Him to heal me until I sense that He tells me to stop. Why would I quit asking, seeking, and knocking when I have not clearly heard Him say no? It is obvious that the help of man and my own self-effort are insufficient. I need God!

It's not that He is absent from the other forms of help—physical therapy and medical intervention. All wisdom is God's. Any good we can accomplish ultimately comes from Him. But, some of this journey is only attributable to His direct hand of involvement.

The lines between these elements are not as clear as I've made them out to be. They blur from day to day. I can't dissect them, and I don't feel the need to attempt to do so. I simply testify that there has been a fascinating interplay between the three.

It causes me to wonder if we don't often have a part to play in our own healing. Please understand. There are some things only God can do and no amount of human effort will ever be sufficient. But, at times, it seems that God looks to us to do our part as well.

While I knew I must lean into prayer and trust God for healing, I should also use every means available to me that He provides. Faith in Him doesn't necessarily mean passivity on our part. Often faith calls more action out of us. Discernment is obviously needed for each situation.

# NO MIRACLE IN SIGHT

As spring arrived, my muscle condition and overall health was still weak and sickly, but had become bearable. I could function with a measure of normalcy. The largest hurdle still to cross—or healing still to be experienced—was my inability to swallow.

My next effort to address this issue led me to Dr. Skarada, an otolaryngologist (more simply known as an ear, nose and throat specialist, or an ENT). He knew my story before I arrived in his office and was eager to see me. He exuded hope as he assured me that he would do everything he could to assist me.

After seeking to understand my case further, he explained that he wanted to run a scope up my nose and follow that path to look at my throat. I must have flinched as he explained the procedure because he quickly added, "I do this to five-year-olds and they don't cry, so you can handle it."

This, of course, was doctor-speak for "Man up, Buddy."

I didn't cry and was actually fascinated by the two minute video he took of the inner workings of my nasal passage and throat.

"You have a deviated septum, but that's common," he explained as he guided the scope.

"Ah, your soft palate isn't closing all the way, that's why you have such nasality in your voice. See that right there? You have about a three millimeter separation. Air is escaping through your nose when you talk rather than coming out of your mouth. It's significant, but I've seen worse."

Down his scope painlessly passed into the region of my throat. He asked me to attempt to swallow. The scope revealed the same verdict as the Modified Barium Swallow Test. The swallow function was non-existent. My esophagus remained closed and inoperable. And, I was about to learn that "inoperable" had a double meaning. Not only did my swallow not function, but there was no operation that could fix it.

Before I knew it, the exam was complete and he gave a surprising summary, "You don't have cancer or trauma. There are no signs of cancer cells or injury in the region. That's actually not as good of news as you might think because there are things I could do to fix those problems. The real problem is that your epiglottis and esophagus aren't functioning."

I was sobered but not surprised by his news.

He closed our lengthy session with a promise that he'd explore what possibilities might be available. He had connections to some of the most respected leaders in the field. He'd share with me his results at our next appointment. Meanwhile, I was to continue to meet with my speech/swallow therapist.

A month later, when I came in for my next appointment, Dr. Skarada was far more subdued. He gave me another guided tour with his scope for good measure, but nothing had changed. His conversations with the experts hadn't produced any hopeful solutions. He could inject my esophagus with Botox to relax the muscle, he explained. But he offered no hope that any long-term benefit would result from the procedure, and I declined.

Later he would acknowledge to me, "If there had been a medical miracle waiting for you at Harvard or Mayo, I would have sent you there. But there was no miracle solution available."

Unknown to me at the time, he consulted with my internal medicine doctor, Dr. Byrkit. Together they agreed that—based on all they knew of my condition—it was unlikely that I'd ever swallow again.

I'm glad that my doctors didn't tell me at the time that they had reached this troubling conclusion. I don't know that my spirit could have born the weight of that news.

What I did know was that this lifestyle was "hard to swallow." I wrote the blog community,

> I'm trying not to keep track of time, but it has been about fifteen months now since I last swallowed. Fifteen months of continual spitting. Fifteen months of smelling food I cannot eat. Fifteen months of pouring cans of "medical food" down my feeding tube. Fifteen months of feeling like an odd ball in a world that eats as they meet, and eats as they walk, and eats as they drive, and eats as they watch TV, and eats as they get up in the morning, and eats before they go to bed, and eats when they celebrate, and eats pretty much whenever they feel like it. And if they aren't eating, they have a cup in their hand. Some days the swallowing of liquid is even a greater craving than eating food. To have my throat quenched with a soothing glass of water, or grape juice, or chocolate milk, or soda—ah, that will be a good day.

God was the only real hope I had that the day would come when I would swallow again. Prayer was my only real strategy. The help of man had been beneficial in some areas, but had reached a disappointing dead end with my inability to swallow.

Add this to my list of the countless reasons I am deeply grateful to be a follower of Christ: My grounds for hope aren't limited to human resources. When everything people can do has failed and our options have run out, our reason to have hope has not. As long as there is a God, we have a basis for hope. And if there is one thing of which I am certain, it is this: We will always have God.

# PART THREE

Give us aid against the enemy,
For the help of man is worthless.
With God we will gain the victory,
And he will trample down our enemies.

*Psalm 108:12-13*

# PREACHING TO MYSELF

"Let's go on a road trip!"

I liked my idea as soon as I said it. There's nothing new about that. The surprising part is that Joanna thought it was a good idea, too.

All the right factors converged for a good road trip. Our older son, Josiah, was soon to graduate from Crown College in Minnesota and we were determined to celebrate with him in person. Many people across the nation continued to pray for us and we wanted to thank them. Our church graciously allowed my vacation time to accumulate, so I had time banked. I was now driving on a daily basis without difficulty, as long as I had my trusty spit cup next to me. It seemed that nothing stood between us and a long trip.

And, frankly, we were restless. Our house—beautiful though it is—played host to countless dark moments and long days. We sensed that a change of scenery would do us good.

The plans came together quickly. My worries that our old minivan wouldn't survive the trip caused me to look into rental cars. I found a great rate for a month long rental. My nephew in Tennessee has a ministry we wanted to see, and he expressed enthusiasm when we mentioned a visit. So it was decided. We would travel from our home in Oregon to the graduation in Minnesota by way of Tennessee. This would be a *real* road trip—thirty days and 7,500 miles.

As we began to pack, we calculated how much feeding tube formula I would need for a month. My diet consisted of seven cans a day. Thus, I would need over 200 cans for the trip. Nine cases of formula consumed most of our trunk space. Our suitcases would have to ride in the backseat.

The morning that we were to leave, I stopped by the church office to take care of a few last details. I always feel better about leaving for a trip if my desk is clean and email inbox empty. The desk and inbox will quickly refill while I'm away, but I can at least have a moment of satisfaction that I'm caught up...fleeting though it is.

With that "I'm going on vacation" feeling, I left the office, got into our rental car, and headed home to pick up Joanna. As I waited at a stoplight, I noticed a cute yellow Volkswagen two cars ahead of me and one lane over.

*Joanna has always liked those VW Bugs. They always come in great colors, too.*

As the light turned green, I watched as the driver of the Volkswagen responded quickly, zipping into the intersection. An instant later, I was shocked to see a Lincoln Town Car enter from the intersecting street. The driver of the Lincoln wasn't going excessively fast, but was clearly running a red light. I winced as he broadsided the rear third of the Volkswagen and sent it into a full spin. The VW finally came to a stop as it slammed against a curb. The driver of the Town Car sat stunned in his relatively undamaged vehicle in the middle of the intersection. The young woman in the VW burst into tears, but appeared to be physically okay. Her car, on the other hand, was not.

By the time I safely parked and walked back, the police had arrived at the accident scene. There were tears, frowns, and worried looks, but no significant injuries. I gave an officer my contact information and reported to him what I witnessed. He took notes of my report and then kindly told me I was free to go.

As I got back into my vehicle, I prayed,

*We've got a lot of miles ahead of us, Lord. Lots of things can happen on the road. I ask you to take care of us, but I'll take this as a reminder that I need to be cautious as well.*

Our first stop was just an hour up the road. Our denomination's annual gathering for district churches was being held in Portland. I was invited to speak for the closing session. My voice was weak, my step unsteady, and my spit rag still in full use, but I was back—at least 140 pounds of me was.

I was happy. It felt so good to be back in circulation. We thanked people for praying for us, reconnected with old friends, and made a few new ones. And I had the joy of doing what I missed so deeply: preach.

I must confess that my message to the conference erupted like a verbal volcano. My sermon was an unkempt barrage of a dozen random points I had been thinking about in my sequestered state. I spewed out my message with all the strength I had. If no one else benefited, I did. Hope was being renewed within me that I would have opportunities to preach again.

Somewhere in the rambling message I talked about the Old Testament character, Joseph. I read,

"They afflicted his feet with fetters, he himself was laid in irons; until the time that his word came to pass, the word of the LORD tested him" (Psalm 105:18-19 NASB).

Until the time finally came—after many years of waiting—that the word Joseph received from the Lord was fulfilled, the word itself became a test.

I have known Joseph's story for a lifetime. I knew he had youthful dreams of significant leadership that were dashed by his brothers' betrayal. I knew that his story turned from bad to worse as he was imprisoned on false charges. I knew that the shackles and chains he wore had the potential of enslaving his spirit as badly as his body.

But the thought that was new for me in this message was that the very word that Joseph had spoken—the word that he *knew* he had heard from God—became the same word that tested him. His trial was difficult enough, but exponentially adding to its harshness was the fact that he had heard from God that he would live a much different life. Until that word from the Lord came to pass, that very message would test him, taunt him.

He believed the word for years. He "preached" the word to his family. Now, his own "sermon" mocked him.

In between uses of my ever present spit rag, I confessed to the audience at the conference that I had experienced something similar. Before becoming ill, I often preached on the goodness of God. Even during recovery, I repeatedly declared that "God is in this and He is good."

But, I admit, when I have dark days and can't see the goodness of God, my own message mocks me. I'm tested by my own words. This is part of the discipleship journey. This is part of God's training.

This also gives me pause about what I preach. I'm increasingly aware that I might have to live out the words I speak in deeper ways than I ever imagined.

I don't know how discouraged Joseph became as he lived for years with an unfulfilled dream. I do know that when his big moment came, his heart was ready. He was just a shave and a change of clothes away from being prepared to stand in the presence of the Pharaoh and receive the promotion of a lifetime (Genesis 41:14, 40).

*Father, please help me live in such a way that I am always ready for what you have next for me.*

I drove away from the conference with two gifts I hadn't had in a long time: an honorarium in my pocket and satisfaction in my heart. Our trip was off to a good start.

# THE OPEN ROAD

Any trip that leads you through the Columbia Gorge of Western Oregon has to be a great trip. As I-84 straddles the majestic Columbia River, a driver like me must be disciplined to not stare too long at the surrounding beauty: the towering trees, mountain views, and Multnomah Falls. Then, it always fascinates me, with just a few bends of the road east of Hood River, the landscape suddenly changes and the temperature rises. The green blanket of the Pacific Northwest has a very narrow fringe. At sixty-five miles per hour, the landscape turns rocky and brown in just a few minutes. Fir trees are replaced by sage brush. The snowy peaks stand guard for vast wheat fields.

For the next two days we traveled on only two roads, I-84 and I-80. I love a trip when the MapQuest directions tell me I don't have to change roads for 764 miles. Find the right exit and drive for another 388 miles.

*This is what I call a road trip. Oregon, Idaho, Utah. Fabulous.*

After a year and a half of traveling in small circles—from home, to the church office, to a doctor's office, and back home again—the open road felt really good. All was well, except that by the time we left Utah, winter had returned for one last visit. The entire state of Wyoming was under a blanket of falling snow. White knuckled drivers fought white out conditions for a 250 mile stretch of ice covered road.

With images of the VW car accident in my mind, I drove through the blizzard at half the speed my Minnesota roots would have prompted me to drive. This was still twice the speed Joanna wanted me to drive. Yes, we argued about it. Yes, we got over it. Yes, we were really glad to get to Cheyenne and turn south out of the storm into Colorado.

Having lived in Colorado Springs in the past, we know too many people to be able to see everyone in the day we had allotted to stay, but the conversations we did have time for were joyful.

*This is exactly why I wanted to take this trip. I'm getting to personally thank these dear friends who have stood by us during this ordeal.*

It was a pleasant Saturday in Colorado Springs. As the afternoon sun tried to re-introduce springtime, Joanna and I sat in its welcoming rays with some friends at a coffee shop. We shared great memories, stories, and laughs. What we couldn't share were the beverage and cookies. As my wife and friends sipped and munched, I poured three cans of formula down my tube...my normal routine. While I envied what they held in their hands, I had at least become accustomed to doing my form of "eating" in public.

On Sunday we made our way to a church outside of Denver. We had never been there before and arrived late. We only knew one person in the church, Jennifer, and I had not seen her in thirty years. Back in our high school days, we served on a Teen Missions team in Haiti. We lost contact with each other through the years, but Jennifer heard the story of my illness and began praying for Joanna and me. She recruited her whole Sunday school class to pray as well. She sent us notes of encouragement and amazingly thoughtful gifts. She had the uncanny ability to find books that I truly benefited from reading. I'm a very picky reader, so her knack is especially surprising.

I had been looking forward to thanking Jennifer personally. What I wasn't prepared for was that her entire Sunday school class of a few dozen young adults had adopted our story. We encountered a whole classroom full of Christians we had never met who were truly excited to see us. Tears came to the eyes of a few of the people as they greeted us. I was surprised and touched by the emotional response from people we didn't know.

In time I came to understand the phenomena. When a person truly prays for someone else, an emotional bond is often formed in the heart of the one praying. The heart of the one praying opens up to the person for whom they are interceding. The storylines of the pray-er and pray-ee start to intermingle.

Again it strikes me,

*The body of Christ is beautiful when she is functioning as Jesus intended!*

After church and the Sunday school class were over, Jennifer and her husband welcomed us to their home for lunch. It was a very pleasant afternoon. The conversation was sweet, but I just have to take their word for the taste of the food.

In her kindness—and as an act of faith—Jennifer set a place for me at the dining room table and explained, "I know you can't swallow, but I thought that maybe today would be the day you could."

I recognized that she was being thoughtful and full of faith, and I kept my response to myself, but I could not help thinking,

*There is no way that I'll swallow today. I don't know if there will ever be a day I'll swallow. I know I will eat in heaven, but I don't know if I will ever eat again on this planet.*

# STUCK IN ST. LOUIS

On Monday, as we traveled through Kansas, Joanna kindly bought me a McDonald's ice cream sundae. I enjoyed tasting and feeling its cold sweetness melt in my mouth. Yet, as always, none of it made its way down my immobile throat, and I was forced to spit it back out.

I hope you never need to know this little safety tip, but I found it better to spit into a cup as I drove than any other method of getting rid of my saliva. I never became completely comfortable with "recreational eating" and so there were many days I "ate" little or nothing. Yet, my saliva production required continuous need for spitting. In the car, rags were cumbersome, paper towels quickly piled up, and opening the car door to spit on the pavement while driving was dangerous. The spit cup was the perfect solution.

The spit cup became my constant driving companion. Joanna took great caution to not grab the wrong cup out of the cup holder between us! At nearly every stop we made, she refilled her Diet Coke and I emptied my spit cup. I never liked to see more than a couple inches of its slithery substance sloshing next to me. I do owe a few businesses across the Midwest an apology for defiling their parking lots. But, hey, the rain washes it away, right?

On Tuesday I woke up to a common sight: a mound of Kleenex next to my bed—evidence of another night of spit-interrupted sleep. We were staying at a hotel in St. Louis. I got out of bed to do my normal routine—read my Bible while pouring some breakfast down my tube.

But on this day, I decided to have something different for breakfast. Eight cases of feeding tube formula still filled our trunk, but the hotel had a free breakfast bar with milk and yogurt—four ounce containers of Yoplait Red Raspberry Yogurt, to be exact. I have poured yogurt thinned with milk down my tube a few times before. Each time, I felt like it made my body happy to not have another meal of formula.

With one hand holding the syringe full of milky yogurt, I opened my Bible to where I left off from the day before: Psalm 108. I poured a few more ounces of breakfast into my tube and continued to read slowly. After so many months of the scripture feeling like sandpaper to my soul, the sweetness of God's Word had returned to me. I wanted to savor the words.

An internal smile arose as I read the final verses of the chapter:

*O grant us help against the foe, for human help is worthless* (Psalm 108:12 New Revised Standard).

I poured a few more ounces into the syringe and thought,

*Yep. I sure need divine help with this "foe." Doctors have done a lot for me, but with my swallowing, human help has been pretty worthless.*

I continued reading,

*With God we shall do valiantly; it is he who will tread down our foes* (Psalm 108:13 NRS).

The verse fascinated me. There it was in the scripture again: We have our part to do in the battle—"we shall do valiantly"—but He is ultimately the one who must be victorious for us—"it is he who will tread down our foes." We are invited into a human/divine partnership. There are some things only God can do. There are some things He expects us to do. We are partners in battle with the victorious God.

*I wonder what my part is in this battle today.*

Somewhere in the midst of this breakfast/devotional time, my feeding tube malfunctioned. It had clogged many times before, so I was not at all concerned at first. A plunger is provided for the feeding tube syringe to deal with clogs.

I placed the plunger in the tube and gave it a gentle push as I had done dozens of times before. Normally, just a small amount of pressure is needed to clear the tube. When the blockage releases, it causes a little "poof" to go off in my stomach, but it's no big deal.

This time, however, my gentle push didn't budge the blockage. I pushed as hard as I could, to no avail. I stood up next to the wall and leaned forward against it, placing all of my weight against the syringe plunger. Nothing moved.

About this time, Joanna returned to the room after finishing her own breakfast. I explained that my tube was stuck and I needed her help. She gave the plunger a little push and was surprised by the resistance. My tube had never acted this way before. We had operated it without any problems since being released from the hospital fifteen months earlier. I told her to go ahead and push as hard as she could.

I felt serious hesitation as I told her to push hard. If a gentle push of the syringe makes a little "poof" in my stomach, what will this syringe full of yogurt do if it suddenly breaks through? I was seated in a desk chair with rollers next to a sliding glass door. As Joanna stood over me, pushing on the plunger as hard as she could, I watched her arm muscles quiver from the effort.

*Oh, boy! If this thing blows it's going to shoot me right out the sliding glass door!*

Instead, I sat motionless in my chair as my feeding tube sat completely stuck. It was inoperable. It didn't appear to be clogged. It appeared to be broken.

*Oh, great! Here I am in a hotel room in St. Louis, half a nation away from my doctors, and my feeding tube quits on me.*

I dumped out the yogurt, pulled out the syringe, and wiped up a few drips that spilled. My Bible still lay open to the same page.

*Human help is worthless. Act valiantly. He treads down our foes.*

I couldn't help but notice the concern on Joanna's face. It was more than concern. It was weariness. She had stood by me so faithfully and cared for me so sacrificially. It was difficult to be the sick one, but the burden the caregiver carries is unique. She had paid a price in this long battle.

We stood in the hotel room, hugged each other, and prayed.

"Lord, why are you withholding the ability to swallow from me?" I asked. Joanna held me tight and affirmed my prayer.

As we packed up our suitcases and checked out of the hotel, Joanna asked me what I was going to do about my tube. My sole source of nutrition, hydration, and medication was not working. Should we find an emergency room before leaving town?

I explained that I wanted to head down the road. There must be plenty of hospitals between St. Louis and Louisville. Besides, I was restless. I wanted to conquer a few miles of the road.

And I wanted more time to pray and think. I hate always using hospitals and doctors as a first response. It seems so "modern," so "American," so "something I don't like" to immediately seek human help. Shouldn't we pray first? Wouldn't it be a good idea to wait a little bit before we came up with our own plan?

Please don't read my response as a "spiritual" one as if I were full of faith at this moment. I wasn't. I was a mix of frustration, confusion, anger, and curiosity.

*What's going on? Why here? Why now? Of all the places my tube could malfunction, why does it have to be here? Where's God in all this? What's with that verse from the Psalms? Was God saying something to me today?*

As Joanna loaded the suitcases—something she did the entire trip because I simply wasn't strong enough to do it—I sent a text message to a few family members.

*In St. Louis. Feeding tube stuck. If God doesn't heal today, I'll have to find an emergency room.*

# STUNNED

My sister, Delores, lives in Indiana. We were looking forward to being with her and her family in a few days. She has a well earned reputation for being a fabulous cook. She was the first to text me back.

*What can we do?*

An answer that startled me immediately came to my spirit:

*Tell her to bake a cheesecake.*

Cheesecake is one of my favorites. Okay, I have a long list of favorites, especially after not eating for so long; but cheesecake ranks way up there on life's pleasure meter.

An argument arose within me:

*Why tell her to bake a cheesecake? No. I'm not going to do that.*

Something within me countered:

*Maybe this is an opportunity to make a declaration of faith that perhaps this is the day that God will heal.*

Fear and faithlessness held me back.

*No.*

Quite simply, I didn't have the faith to believe that in a few days I'd be eating cheesecake. Looking back, I'm convinced that God's Spirit was whispering words of faith to me, but I rejected them. I had prayed so many times—so many people had prayed so many times—that my ability to swallow would be restored. Nothing had happened. Why get my hopes up now?

I texted my sister back the "Christian" response.

*Pray.*

Again, looking back, I believe I can see more clearly what was happening. The "Christian" response of asking for prayer was at that moment a very "un-Christian" thing to do. To be a Christian—to be like Christ—is to obey God. God was calling me to take a step of faith—to ask my sister to do something she would have been thrilled to do, bake one of her specialties for her brother who hadn't eaten in seventeen months. Instead of taking a step of faith, I stalled. So much for acting valiantly.

I know that this point I'm making could easily confuse some. I want to be careful how I make it. Yet, I've come to believe that as vital as prayer is, as central as it is to our walk with God and His work in our lives, as pivotal as it is for our intimate relationship with Him; there are times that prayer can become a cop-out. When God is clearly calling us to take a step of faith, to act in some way, I don't think He's too excited when we sit around and talk about it some more...even if we're talking to Him.

Certainly we can pray *while* we are obeying. We can pray *and* act at the same time. But, there are times we must get off of our knees, back onto our feet, and do something about what we've been praying about.

I want to be an advocate for prayer. I want to be an example of prayer. Yet, I pray that I'll never use prayer as an excuse for not doing what God is calling me to do.

I wasn't thinking any of this as I made my way out of the city on I-64 and into the farmlands of Illinois. Instead, I was thinking about what I had read in Psalm 108. I was thinking about Joanna as she sat next to me in the passenger's seat with tears streaming down her face. I imagined that she looked like Hannah of Samuel's day, tearfully interceding in silence.

And, I was thinking about the two four ounce containers of Yoplait Red Raspberry Yogurt in my backpack. I had taken these extra containers from the breakfast bar with the intent of pouring them down my tube. With my tube stuck, they remained unused and unopened.

When it seemed appropriate, I asked Joanna to get one out and open it for me. Over our many road trips through the years, I had enjoyed snacking as I drove. Being unable to swallow obviously made this impossible. But, today I could at least enjoy the taste of the yogurt and then spit it into my ever-waiting cup in the holder next to me.

Joanna found a spoon and fed me a tiny bite. The thought came to me,

*You have a part in this. Don't spit.*

As the miles passed, I repeatedly tried to get the first bite of yogurt to go down. Getting it out of my mouth was easy enough, but as always, it seemed to just sit in the back of my throat.

*Don't spit. You have your part in this.*

Repeatedly, I brought it up from my throat, back into my mouth and tried again. I asked Joanna for another small bite, and then another.

*Is it happening? Could it really be happening?*

Like a flower bud slowly opening it's petals to the sun, my stuck esophagus seemed to be slowly awakening. It was almost imperceptible at first. I was skeptical.

*Maybe I'm just imagining this. Maybe the yogurt is sitting down there in the recesses of my throat.*

So many prayers had seemed to go unheeded. So many days of silence had been lived. A miracle was happening, but I was slow to accept it and said nothing to Joanna about it for seventy-five miles.

Eventually I asked Joanna to look into the yogurt container. It had gone down one ounce.

"So?"

"I haven't spit yet."

Hope and faith instantly leapt in our hearts. We, who had prayed together countless times, now prayed with a hope and intensity we had never experienced. She reached over and placed her hand on my throat, something she had done so many times before. We both prayed.

Mile post after mile post passed, but they were invisible to me. My wife was interceding for me. I was caught up in my prayers and hers. Sometimes I could understand her words and sometimes I couldn't, her words choked by her emotion. Streams of tears ran down both our faces.

She reached over again to touch my throat as she prayed. This time I felt a slight movement in the area of my throat that had been motionless for so long.

*It's happening! It's really happening!*

In my raspy voice, I started to sing an old song. It's not a song I've ever liked all that much, but it seemed to be the word for the moment,

*In the name of Jesus, in the name of Jesus,*
*We have the victory.*

Then I tried a small sip of orange juice. It went down. I was stunned! I knew from my experiences with the speech/swallow therapists that liquids were especially difficult and dangerous because they can so quickly slip down into the windpipe. Just the night before I sampled a swig of soda, only to have it immediately rejected by my unwilling throat. Now, just fourteen hours later, I swallowed juice. The dozens of muscles and nerves that need to work in cooperation for the swallow to function were awakening from their long slumber.

A tiny, tiny burp arose. Like a small lone bubble coming up from the silence of a lake floor, I felt it rise to the surface. I could feel the little wisp of air climb the once lifeless corridor. Who knew that a burp could be so hope-giving? A part of my body was coming alive again and I could feel it!

By the time we reached Grayville, Illinois, I had swallowed two ounces of yogurt. I texted the family and called our church with the news. We pulled over at a Casey's Convenience Store. Casey's was offering free cookie samples—one sixth of a macadamia nut cookie. I took a small bite of it, chewed it cautiously, and gulped…and then gulped again. It went down! Who ever thought that a cheap convenience store cookie could bring such delight? I went back to the car almost in a daze. Was this really happening? Was God really healing me?

Joanna and I stood by the car in the gas station parking area, held each other, and declared God's goodness.

I began to proclaim: "You have been healing me, You are healing me, You will heal me!"

And then, "Greater is He that is in me than he that is in the world. Greater is He that is in me than he that seeks to destroy. Greater is He that is in me than the disease that is in me. Greater is He that is in me than anything that is against me."

I then took my spit cup, and as an act of faith, walked over to the garbage can and threw it away. By God's grace, I was starting a new era.

# GETTING TO THE BOTTOM OF IT

Joanna drove as we left Grayville and headed further east. I kept trying to eat. We pulled off the freeway into a rest area. I sat and stared at a sight I could barely comprehend. I was looking at the bottom of an empty four ounce yogurt container.

*Where did it go? Did I actually eat all of that? After so long, could it be true?*

I believe I was in a mild state of shock. It was happening! The miracle was happening! All those prayers were finally being answered. All those months of wondering if anything would ever change were suddenly coming to an end.

I got out of the car, stopped the first guy I saw, and handed him my camera. He's probably still wondering why he took a picture of a guy with a goofy grin holding an empty yogurt container while standing next to his red-eyed wife. I didn't try to explain.

We drove farther, sang more, prayed more, and nibbled more. After about four hours, I recorded that I had eaten one third of a banana with now a total of six ounces of yogurt. It wasn't easy. There were times I was tempted to spit. I determined not to. I kept reminding myself that I had a part in this process.

A couple coughing fits served warning that the dozens of muscles and nerves required for a successful swallow were still unaccustomed to working together and that food doesn't automatically go down the right pipe. I definitely wasn't swallowing normally, yet...but by the kindness of God I was swallowing!

Matching the pleasure of eating was the fact that for the first time since my hospitalization, I had no demanding need to spit. The "spit or drown" sensation I had lived with 24/7 was gone and never returned. My abandoned spit cup was never needed again.

As we continued to drive east into Indiana, we saw a sign for an historic site: The Lincoln Boyhood National Memorial, Abe's early home just ten minutes off I-64. Lincoln is one of Joanna's favorite historic figures and so we stopped.

As Joanna toured the visitor center and site of the cabin, I sat in the car under the shade of a fabulous grove of trees. I pulled out my laptop to capture some of the events and emotions of the day. I recorded,

"A few ounces of yogurt and a swig of juice don't usually lead to great celebration, but today it did! It was the evidence we needed that God was stepping in on this day...the very day my tube ceased to function. All through this journey of sickness, God has shown His sovereignty through timing. Once again He did so. On the morning my tube died, my throat came to life. Amazing!"

After leaving the Memorial, our next stop was Wendy's. I ordered the biggest Frosty they make. Chocolate. While just the day before, the ice cream Joanna bought for me sat rejected in the back of my lifeless throat, now I had the pleasure of feeling the cold of that Frosty go all the way down.

*Wow.*

I remembered back to the last Frosty I had unsuccessfully tried so many months earlier on our way home from rehab. I remembered all the lonely times of not being able to join people for the pleasure of a meal. I remembered the envy of seeing other people with a cup in their hand.

But now I mostly just sipped, and savored...and swallowed.

*Thank you, Jesus. Thank you. Thank you, Jesus. Thank you. Thank you, Jesus.*

It took me four hours to drink that Frosty—about the same time as my slowest marathon. This was a "marathon" of pleasure.

Sometime after dark, we arrived at our hotel in Tennessee. I plugged in my laptop and as I made my way slowly through a cup of Wendy's chili, I shared our happy news with the world via our blog. I couldn't think of anything witty or profound, so I simply titled the entry, "Rejoice with Me."

With happy taste buds and a happier heart, I did my best to reflect on the amazing events of the day. I wanted others to share my joy and praise our God. As I savored the last bites of chili, I concluded my post:

> I have so many lessons to share…so much of God to reflect on… so many calories to try to consume so that I can appropriately leave the feeding tube behind; but for this moment, I just want to celebrate and I want you to do so with me.
>
> To the hostess who believed for me this week when I couldn't; thank you! To the brother in Oklahoma who has fasted from ice cream on my behalf for the duration of this ordeal; your commitment is complete. Have a big bowl…with toppings! To the parents whose children have prayed for me with unusual regularity; throw a "Yay, Jesus" party! Don't miss this teaching/celebrating opportunity. To all of you friends…literally scattered across the globe… bring glory to God. A God-timed miracle took place today. You were part of it. Thank Him!

By Facebook and phone and a flurry of other communication, the news spread literally around the world. This was again evidence of the beauty of the body of Christ on our behalf. In the next days, thousands of people would log onto the blog to read the story for themselves. Hundreds of people—lifelong friends and "prayer friends" we had never met—made comments.

# JOY MULTIPLIED

Great news, answers to prayer, and a joyful heart are fantastic in themselves. But when the celebration is shared by others, it triples our pleasure. Joy kept to ourselves never feels completely satisfying. Reading the comments that poured in made our joy complete. This is a small sampling of the comments we received:

> Praise God!! The wonderful news is spreading around Facebook quickly!! I cried tears of joy and praise as I read your blog this morning!! Today is our daughter's 11th birthday, and tonight when we go to Baskin-Robbins to celebrate, it's gonna be a "Yay Jesus" party too!!!! We love you Pastor John! What a MIGHTY GOD WE SERVE!!!!
>
> #9 J., M., R., J., S. & J.

> John and Joanna
>
> Praise the Lord. When I read the news last night I hurried to tell my husband, even if I had to wake him up. Praise the Lord, the Great Healer. This is truly an answer to many, many prayers and done in His time. May this encourage you that continued healing is to come and God will bless you richly.
>
> #13 D. & K. R.

> John, I read a quick note on Facebook about you swallowing and had to come here to see if was true. YES, YES, YES it is true, you are swallow-

---

ing. I am totally crying as I write this. God is good, He is good indeed. I know this is a painful journey for you and your family, but rest assured, we hurt when you hurt, we rejoice when you rejoice. PRAISE GOD. I have my radio on now and Delirious is playing "Did you feel the mountains tremble." YES, I did and do. Love you man, may God continue to bless you and all you do for Him.

#18 J. F.


PRAISE GOD!!!! Our family has been praying for you daily—all our boys included—trusting and believing that God would answer this prayer for your ability to swallow. I couldn't even read your blog out to our boys this morning without stopping to control my tears at many points. GOD IS GOOD, GOD IS GOOD. There is rejoicing in our house today. ...And there are three boys who have just seen firsthand what God does in response to persistent prayer. Thank you so much for sharing this journey with all of us—so honestly and regularly. God is using you and your experience in a mighty way.

#27 K. R.


John & Joanna,

We are praising the Lord & celebrating the great news!!! Yay, Jesus, Yay, Jesus, Yay, Jesus!!! We have shared tears, numerous phone calls & shouts for joy!!! The first thing our four year old said was "Yay, John Stumbo can swallow! When are we having hot cocoa & brownies? Can we have our party today?" We are jumping for joy and praising God.

What a day! What a wonderful day for a miracle!

*And Nehemiah continued, "Go and celebrate with a feast of rich foods and sweet drinks, and share gifts of food with people who have nothing prepared. This is a sacred day before our Lord. Don't be dejected and sad, for the joy of the LORD is your strength!"* (Nehemiah 8:10 NLT)

Big Celebration hugs to you both!

Much Love,

#57 C., T. A., A., A., & A.


Celebrating with tears flowing! Please pass the Kleenex!

#58 J.

Dear John and Joanna, Unlike the joyful dancers out there and those looking up favorite brownie recipes, I am frozen in awe. I keep quietly relishing this phenomenal miracle. I am so grateful for this precious, merciful act of God, and I'm treasuring the detailed words of your prayers, cries, and spiritual, hands-on warfare. Thank you for taking the time to write to describe your pleading and praying as you were experiencing your swallow grow. It is such a privilege to pray on your behalf. Complete healing Jesus!!! Praise praise praise!

#78 L. W.


WOW!!! I read it first on Twitter and then checked in with staff at church to make sure what I was reading wasn't a falsehood.... AMAZING! A miracle of epic God proportions! Glory and honor and praise to Him. Powerful. I love what He has done and is doing and will continue to do through your life. Beautiful.

#84. S. R.


We got word of your swallowing via a 1:30 AM text. Someone who was so excited that they couldn't sleep felt we should share in her 1:30 AM joy as well. The news was so worth being awakened for! We were praising God in the middle of the night and have continued to do so throughout the day as we have thought about your news.

#86. C. & S.


This is the best news ever!!!! Oh how we've waited with you for this day. Can't imagine the tears that were shed as everyone read this blog entry. I sure cried my portion way over here in Iraq. It is surely a miracle from our merciful God. You TWO have made a mark on me in ways you'll never know. Thank you thank you, Jesus!

#90 C. P.


I'm wondering if people who don't know what's going on are wondering why there are so many people wandering around with goofy grins and tears rolling down their cheeks! How wonderful to be among those who are rejoicing over the miracle! Praise Him indeed!

#98 N. T.

Dear John and Joanna,

I have been a silent but loyal and grateful student at the John and Joanna Stumbo Seminary. Only eternity will tell the effect of your transparent journey of faith and fidelity. I certainly add my strongest Amen to the great cloud of witnesses praising our God for this wonderful news.

#137 D. C.


Ever since I heard the great news I've been singing the Doxology! I love you both dearly & I will see you soon.

#140 M. (John's ninety-year-old mother)


I'm so happy for you and praising the Lord with you! Tears are flowing in Costa Rica!! I would love to hear the list of every single thing you eat for the next few weeks! John, you have been such an encouragement to me in the last year. I haven't made any comments on your blog, but I've read every single thing you've written and you have been such a blessing to me. Like so many other people have said, there aren't words to express my joy for the mere fact that you can eat food!

#148 R.


CHILLS!!! And a heart full of gratitude to God for this gift for you! I feel like singing . . .

Big, big hug,

#167 A. C.


John and Joanna,

Can I just say how excited and happy I am for you! I went snowboarding Tuesday morning with a couple friends and had been talking about you on the way up—explaining a healing story I had heard earlier this year, thinking about you guys—hoping that would be you one day, John. On the way back from the mountain, we got a text from a friend about the amazing news! When I got home, I was asked how snowboarding was—literally my first words out of my mouth were "John Stumbo can swallow, isn't that great!!!" I think I texted my whole contact list in my phone, to share the good news. I'm so incredibly happy for you two. Free steaks on me! Go big or go home, right?

#168 K. S.

With good reason, a friend of mine, Peter, dubbed this experience: The "Swallow Heard 'Round the World." In a world where so many people suffer or celebrate alone, we have been overwhelmed by the fact that so many, many Christ-followers stood by us.

And no one could possibly have stood by me more faithfully than Joanna did. I want you to read her perspective of this remarkable experience.

# THE ROAD TRIP
## *FROM JOANNA'S PERSPECTIVE*

As we left on our road trip, I felt better than I had in a long time. I was ready for a change and have always enjoyed having my family trapped in the car with me for long trips. We planned to see many friends and family along the way, and best of all, we were going to spend several days with just our kids at a lake house in northern Minnesota.

Yet, in spite of the promised pleasures, a dark cloud continued to hover over us. John's inability to eat was a grief we couldn't escape. At home I tried to eat apart from him, but that clearly wouldn't be possible in the car. He would smell and hear every bite I took, unless I quickly went in and ate at a fast-food place, which wasn't much comfort to him either. I knew I had shared many pieces of his pain on this mysterious journey, but I fully understood that in this huge way I could not begin to feel his pain. He complained very little, but I could see how isolated he felt by not being able to swallow.

Our trip got off to a good start as it was fun to see friends at the District Conference. Hearing John preach again was a special highlight. But by the time we got to Wyoming, things turned stressful. Due to a couple accidents when I was young, I'm a very nervous passenger in the snow. Meanwhile, in my opinion, John can be an overly confident driver (some would use the word "aggressive") in the snow. By sundown we made it through the stress of the day. We soon realized that the snow wasn't the only thing we were leaving behind in our rearview mirror.

Then came the morning of April 27. I can only imagine the anticipation we would have felt had we known what this day held for us. But we *didn't* know, and the day's start was anything but exciting. After breakfast, I came into the room and found John with his Bible and his feeding tube, a common sight in the mornings. He asked for my help as something had apparently become stuck in the tube. This was nothing new, but as I tried and tried to push the syringe's plunger, it wouldn't budge. *This* was new as I had always been able to make it work before. I remember John telling me to push as hard as I could, which made me nervous, but I went for it. Again, nothing.

After repeated attempts, I tried to figure out where we could go in a strange city to get help with a clogged feeding tube. In my opinion, John's most urgent need was for his daily medication (we always disagreed on the subject of medications). He would also soon need water and his formula. I was disappointed and frustrated that we would probably have to spend a big chunk of the day in an emergency room, but understood when John suggested we go down the road a bit before we stopped to find one. Maybe something would dissolve or dislodge in the tube if we waited a bit.

The weather was as gloomy as my mood. I was especially disappointed because we had planned for this to be a day when we could take our time as we traveled and visit some historical sites. With the need to stop at an emergency room, this plan seemed unlikely. As we headed down the road I started reading my Bible. I was in 1 Samuel 1, reading about Hannah. Year after year, she had wept and begged God for a child. What was different about the year God finally answered her prayer? Was it the promise she made? Was it simply a matter of God's timing? As we rode I tried to piece her story together with ours and, like Hannah, begged God for healing. I began to cry and pray quietly. I felt deeply sad and almost hopeless. I'm sure John was praying as well, and as we rode on, sometimes we prayed aloud and sometimes quietly alone.

This little prayer service went on for a while and then John asked for a yogurt to eat "recreationally." I obliged and continued to read and pray. Knowing there is power in Jesus' name we began to voice as many of His names as we could think of: "Great Physician, King of Kings, Good Shepherd, Prince of Peace." On and on we went.

We rebuked Satan, we sang praise songs, we begged God, we cried. None of this was new—we had done all of these things before. We had been prayed for by many groups and individuals in many different places. Inspired by the persistent knocking neighbor in Jesus' parable, we weren't ready to give up. And how glad I am that we didn't. For as we cried and prayed, God reached down from the unseen into our rental car and healed John's throat muscles. I watched in stunned joy as he ate bite after bite of yogurt without spitting a drop out! My husband was eating for the first time in a year and a half! It would have been almost unbelievable had it not been so easy to see!

My joy for John was exceptional that day and for many days thereafter. But I believe that my joy in experiencing God's clear and loving intervention on our behalf was every bit as profound. Having John eat again has changed our lives on many levels. I think we'll always appreciate holidays and even simple meals together to a new degree.

But beyond the physical healing, God gently reminded me that just because He hadn't answered sooner, He hadn't abandoned us or coolly turned His back to us. It simply hadn't been the right time. I know He was as happy to heal John on April 27 as we were to have him healed. I also believe that "The LORD, the LORD, the compassionate and gracious God" (Exodus 34:6) had grieved with us for John's pain. How could a loving Father not? But in His complete understanding that's so far beyond mine, He knew that the best day for John to swallow would be that day. And on a much deeper level I trust His wisdom and His power. Most of all, I trust His loving heart.

# MY TUBE AND EATETH, TOO

*No way. I can't believe it!*

I woke up in our Tennessee hotel room in disbelief. I looked around. Next to my pillow and on the floor beside my bed there wasn't a single spit rag or paper towel. I had slept through the night for the first time in this long journey without having to spit.

*Thank you, Jesus!*

If the food I had consumed the previous day wasn't evidence enough, my ability to swallow my saliva in the night was now my final proof that a miracle had indeed occurred. The 24/7 need to spit had been so oppressive for me. I was embarrassed in public, weary in private, and restless all night. But a new day had truly dawned. I woke up from a night of sleep refreshed—a very rare occurrence—and excited over a simple fact: I could eat breakfast!

I was disappointed to find that the breakfast bar of this hotel didn't have a very healthy selection. I hoped for yogurt. Instead, I got biscuits and gravy. I didn't complain, though. For so long I had been cut off from the world of eating that I was happy to reenter it, even if it wasn't my favorite cuisine.

Soon we were off to spend the day with my nephew, Vince, and his delightful family. They are intentionally choosing to live and raise their family in a community that most people would avoid. The use of banned substances and the misuse of alcohol and prescription drugs dominate and decimate the population. Sadness walks the streets. Hopelessness hangs in the air. Apathy slouches in the shadows.

As we drove to Vince's house, we couldn't help but notice that from their exterior appearance, the businesses that seem to best thrive in town are the funeral homes. Death seems to be the dominant theme in this town.

But just on the edge of town, an oasis of life awaits. Vince's family—bursting with energy, smiles, and hugs—welcomed us. We toured, hiked, laughed, and ate with them throughout the day. I felt proud of my nephew as it became obvious to me that he is the unofficial community chaplain. Vince and his delightful wife Misty believe that Jesus truly can make a difference in an individual life and the life of a whole community. As they go about working and raising their family in this setting, they are quiet lovers and leaders of a broken populace. I doubted that I would be willing to make such a sacrifice.

Meanwhile, wherever we went, I ate. I ate all day. The banana was pretty nasty by the time I finished it four hours later. The chocolate shake separated into a watery mixture as the Tennessee heat conquered it before I did. Some orange juice, a few bites of Joanna's enchilada, and a half dozen Pringles rounded out the day. Whether thirsty or not, I took sips from every drinking fountain we passed—just because I could!

By late afternoon, however, I was growing concerned. It was obvious that my new ability to swallow was not sufficient to meet my body's needs. Hydration was a particular concern. I didn't yet have the physical ability to drink a sufficient quantity and with my feeding tube inoperable, I was beginning to feel faint.

Vince is employed as the Human Resources Director for the local hospital, so I knew I had access to medical help if I needed it, but I wasn't done trying on my own quite yet. We tried various times throughout the day to get my feeding tube to work. At one point, I poured a few ounces of Joanna's Diet Pepsi in the tube to see if it would dissolve whatever might be blocking the flow. I had heard stories of cola's power to dissolve things, couldn't it clear my tube? No luck. Further efforts to force water through were ineffective.

Finally, I asked Vince if he had pliers that could cut through wire. He found the proper tool and I showed him where I wanted him to snip. My feeding tube had come specially equipped with an on/off valve. The little red and blue valve was a convenience, making the operation of the tube easier for Joanna and me, but wasn't essential to the functioning of the tube.

Joanna was skeptical about my idea. It is her job to be skeptical. Her cautious skepticism has kept me out of trouble many times in our marriage. I would be a wealthier man if I had listened to her skepticism at certain times in my life. She doesn't call it skepticism. She calls it intuition. You might even be tempted to label it wisdom.

However, on this rare occurrence, I was the one who was right. With a hand as steady as a surgeon, one snip was all it took for Vince to remove the valve. I held the severed piece up to the light and looked through it.

"Aha. See that?! It's clogged!"

I found a toothpick and started to dig.

"Look at this!"

Tiny seeds—red raspberry seeds—Yoplait Yogurt red raspberry seeds—reluctantly gave up their home in my valve. Suddenly it all made sense to me. Being the fiscally conservative guy that I am—Joanna thinks "cheap" might be a better word—I always purchased the lower cost off-brands of yogurt where one doesn't have to contend with the seeds of real fruit. Yoplait, on the other hand, uses a generous quantity of raspberries and not even Diet Pepsi is a match for the power of a pack of raspberry seeds.

My feeding tube was now two inches shorter, but was fully operable again. I gave myself a long "drink" of water and poured in a 300 calorie can of formula for good measure. Immediately, I felt better. I benefited from the hydration and nutrition, but the greater relief came knowing that I not only had dodged going to the hospital, but I could re-enter the world of eating and drinking at a reasonable rate. Rather than needing to go from zero to one hundred percent self-sustaining in one day, I could take my time. After being in disuse for so long, the many little muscles involved in the swallowing process needed some time to rebuild.

I tried to finish the night off with a scoop of ice cream, but after two days of almost non-stop workouts, my swallow muscles let me know in their tiny muscular way that they were tired. I gave them the night off, knowing that there was plenty of ice cream awaiting me in the months ahead.

# LARGE SERVINGS OF GLORY

We reluctantly said good-bye to my nephew's embracing family, and turned our car westward. Indiana was our next stop. My sister, Delores, and her family were waiting for us. And, yes, so was a cheesecake…and fudge and corn soup and lots of other good food. Her cooking seemed to give my system a necessary jump start. The 140 pound body for so long swimming around in my clothes, now suddenly recognized what I was feeding it. It was as if my body said, "I know what to do with that!" After five joyful days in Indiana, I happily announced that I gained "a pound a day at Delores'!"

The weight gain brought with it a gradual increase in strength and energy. We celebrated Josiah's college graduation with great pleasure. A few days in a lakefront cabin in Minnesota became the happiest family times we have had in a few years. The cold and wet weather only served to keep us indoors together. Joanna and I cherished these hours. And for me, every day was a new taste sensation. My wife's cooking, yes! Snack foods, yes! Real fruit, yes! Hot chocolate, yes! Any chocolate, yes!

Meanwhile, stories continued to pour in of people who heard our news. Our sense of celebration was being shared by so many. It was fun, truly fun—a word we rarely used in the past year and a half—to hear of happy dances breaking out in people's homes, tears being shed, Tweets and treats being shared, fasts ended, and praises lifted. The faith of young and old alike was being enlarged, and in the process God was receiving large servings of glory. This made us truly happy.

As we continued to drive west and make our way back to Oregon, Joanna and I had uninterrupted time to process the recent events. The sweetness of what God had been doing only became richer for us. We were struck again by the timing of the events. Not only did God release my lifeless throat on the very day that my feeding tube was stuck, He did so in the "sequestered" location of a rental car in a section of the country where we didn't know a soul.

It was sweet to us that God healed me in a setting where the moment was shared privately between Joanna and me. We were prayed for in public so many times, God could have easily healed me with dozens of praying people gathered around. Often I envisioned myself being healed while on the platform preaching. Wouldn't that have made a great video?

Yet, most of this long journey was traveled with only the two of us side-by-side. And, again, we found a certain sweetness in the fact that we, who shared so many dark hours alone together, now shared a miracle alone together. It has been a precious, tender, and soul-binding experience. There's no one with whom we would have rather shared the miracle.

It also became sweet to us that God healed me in a setting and manner where no one could get glory for it but God alone. Since it was just the two of us inside the confines of a car on a lonely stretch of highway, the spotlight stayed on God—not on some group of elders or gathering of people. No human got in the way of God's glory, which easily could have happened had the miracle occurred in a different setting. The fact that God's glory had no competitors in this experience brought us pleasure.

Joanna and I are quick to acknowledge that on the topic of God's glory we are very limited in our understanding. We feel like lightweights dealing with something so weighty. Yet, our spirits are jealous for this truth to be more fully understood and enjoyed by ourselves and others. We have come to see that the world functions at its best when God is truly glorified. When He is the center of our attention and the sole recipient of our praise, when He is unquestionably obeyed and unreservedly worshipped, when He has captured our affections and consumed our imagination, something "other worldly" happens. Heaven intersects with earth.

We often pray, "Thy Kingdom come, thy will be done on earth as it is in heaven." This prayer—taught to us by Jesus—communicates a longing that earth would come into alignment with heaven. We pray with Jesus that what happens in heaven would happen here on earth—that earth would function as does heaven.

When we find ourselves—through some moment of genuine worship or act of self-forgetful service—entering into the glory-giving, we're doing the very thing for which we were created. We exist—our ultimate purpose in creation is—to bring glory to God. When we do, even for a fleeting moment, the Lord's Prayer is being answered. This is the way heaven always operates. Heaven is perfect because God is always the one receiving the glory. No created being gets in the way of the Creator, but rather each one reflects His greatness.

Joanna and I want our daily lives to be more and more lived for His glory and reflect His glory. There is an alignment, a centering, an "all-is-wellness" to any moment where all allegiance, all affection, and all attention flow to God and God alone. Something leaps in our hearts at that moment—something heavenly, something divine. For a fleeting moment we see a shimmer of what it's like to be in heaven, or at least a foreshadowing of it.

As the aroma arising from an oven promises great things to come, so the feelings that arise in our caged spirits alert us to what awaits at heaven's table.

Does not something or Someone within our spirit testify to us at that moment?

*For this we were created. For this we exist—to bring glory to God.*

Presently, we are small and frail creatures. We cannot sustain this level of focus for long, if we ever attain it at all. But—great news!—we will not always be this weak. Someday we will be large and strong enough to dwell in His glory. Worship in heaven will not be a forced, dutiful activity. We'll be caught, captured, catapulted, and caressed in the experience. It won't just be momentary. We won't have to try to cling to it, and we won't grow weary in it.

With good cause we sing:

*When we've been there ten thousand years*
*Bright shining as the sun*
*We've no less days to sing God's praise*
*Than when we first begun.*

Our current, shriveled capacity to experience the divine will burst open as a sprout breaks out of a seed. Life emerges! We'll grow and grow toward the Son. Vitality will flow where we once only knew death. Our capacity to experience God and participate in the glory-giving will expand far beyond our current imagination. As mortality gives way to immortality, so will our current limitations be overcome.

Heaven will be awe-full. Glory. Glory! Glory!! God's and God's alone! No competitors. No imitators. No distracters. His name will be spoken—countless forms of His name in countless languages. We will have long experiences where His name and none other will burst from our hearts, pour over our voices, and flow like a tributary into a grand river of celebration. Presently, our momentary excursions into glory-giving allow us to feel the passing mist of heaven's continuous waterfall. Someday we'll be strong enough to stand under the full force of its cascading energy. It will be powerful. It will be beautiful. It will be—literally—heavenly.

# WHO IS HE?

Sixteen states and as many beds, a half dozen churches and half a nation of friends, more than a few chocolate shakes, and 8,750 miles later, we were home safely. The road trip had consumed more miles than we expected, but I had consumed far less formula than we ever imagined.

As we re-entered life in Salem, we sensed that change was taking place on multiple levels. We didn't know where it would lead, but with renewed hope we kept praying together for God's guidance for what He had for us next.

I often said to God, *You had plenty of opportunity to take me home to heaven. You must have left me here for a reason. What is it?*

I never became accustomed to that emaciated fellow occupying my house or stumbling along the pier. I looked in the mirror once in a while to find that he was still there, but I never wanted to get to know him. He had a pretty good sense of humor, but other than that, I didn't like having him around. I never invited him in the first place. He could barely smile and walk, he couldn't eat or run, he sighed and groaned a lot—he was actually quite a pain to have around.

But as we resumed life in Salem and summer wore on, I was slowly starting to look, sound, and feel a bit more like "me" again. I continued to gradually gain weight and strength. I was even awarded a speeding ticket—further evidence that I was getting back to my old self.

I was grateful for the renewal of body and spirit I was experiencing. Joanna and I took long summer evening walks, often followed by a

Dairy Queen sundae. I continued my role as an associate pastor on staff at the church I had once led. We were once again in the city, home, and church that we knew so well, but everything looked different now.

One day I needed to be part of a meeting of church leadership. It was a good meeting. It was a necessary meeting. It was a meeting I had often led myself. But on this particular day, as I sat in the meeting, I—without forethought—found myself writing a sentence on the top of the blank sheet of paper that lay before me.

*Did I come back from my deathbed for this?*

I was surprised by my own question. In years past, I would have taken the meeting and my participation in it for granted. I was in leadership. Leaders have meetings. I'd be there. But now, through the vantage point of having been to death's door and back, I found myself analyzing life differently.

*I don't know how many years I have left; do I want to spend them this way? Did God spare my life to sit here and do this?*

The distinction between my own thoughts and God's Spirit speaking to me is sometimes unclear to me. But on this occasion, I did sense that the Spirit of God was gently nudging me. I don't remember the specific words, but the general message to my spirit was, *This is good work. This is necessary work. This work is for someone to do. But is it for* you *to do?*

Meanwhile, as I questioned my own role, I could sense that my presence at church caused confusion for others as well. As my body and voice grew stronger, the question grew in people's minds as to what was next for me.

I found myself often thinking, *There is a reason that lead pastors don't stick around a church after they are done being lead pastors. Their presence complicates things.*

I could tell that my presence was complicating matters for the congregation and some of the staff. More personally, I was having a hard time finding my new niche. When was it appropriate for me, as the ex-leader, to speak and when was it not? What should I do with my occasional concerns? Just because things were different now didn't mean that they weren't good. Things were just different. Could I adjust? Should I adjust? Maybe I was internally striving because I no longer fit. Was this okay?

A wide array of emotions sloshed around within us as we concluded that our time in Salem must come to a close. Without any idea of what might be next for us, we began to take the necessary steps to prepare for a transition: meet with a realtor, list our home, have a garage sale, begin conversations with church leadership about our future, etc.

It sounds contradictory to say it, but my confidence had never been so strong and never so unsteady at the same time. Joanna and I remained convinced that God kept me alive for a reason. We figured that His plan for us would also include some way of keeping a roof over our heads and paying for our expenses. We were more confident than ever in His care.

Meanwhile, my personal confidence had been rattled.

*Can I still lead like I once did? Will anyone take seriously a preacher with a voice that sounds like Red Green? Have I lost my "edge"—whatever that is?*

It didn't help that some months earlier, as I had sat in the office of a potential employer—a ministry that had previously sought to hire me— the president of the organization looked at me sympathetically. Joanna and I could tell that he had no confidence that the skinny guy with a feeding tube hanging from his stomach was fit to lead anything of significance. The conversation was kind but went nowhere.

Neither did it help that a "head hunter" organization that had eagerly sought my resume prior to my getting sick now held me at arm's length. They stated, in so many words, that I was now damaged goods. I was told, *some ministries may see your recent health crisis as an asset, but others won't take a look at you.*

We never heard from the organization again, and we were okay with that. Rattled, as I've said, in our own confidence, we were re-assured that God was up to something. As our house sat on the market month after month without an offer and hardly even a looker, and as the path before us was only clear one or two steps at a time, we took turns encouraging each other. God wasn't done. We would be okay. I was frequently reminded of a sermon I had preached many years before:

> Just because we can't see His hand, just because we can't decipher His plan, doesn't mean that He's not at work. He's the God who is always at work on our behalf, but He doesn't owe us a play-by-play report of what He is doing.

I knew in my spirit that He was giving us another opportunity to trust Him.

*Who am I? What have I become? What does God have next for us? How do I best use my life for Him?*

These questions—and many more like them—roamed like a herd of elk through my mind. Most of the questions remain unanswered. Answers are often overrated anyway. Our God desires for us to seek Him, and few things inspire the search for Him quite like unanswered questions.

Who is this guy looking at me in the mirror? Some days, I'm still not sure. But I am more certain than ever that Someone else is involved—deeply involved—in my story.

# SAME HOUSE, NEW FOUNDATION

The conversation won't go away. It is over a year old, but keeps coming up in my head. As a friend of mine stood at my hospital bedside, fully believing that I would someday recover, he asked, "What are you going to leave behind?"

"Huh?" I didn't pick up on his thought at first pass.

"You've been through something so traumatic; it would be a shame to waste the experience by coming out of it as the same guy who went into it. What do you want to leave in the past?"

I had no real answer for him at the time. Yet, his question lingers with me over the many months.

In time it becomes clear that one significant piece to leave in the past is my tendency to dishonor my wife. For some seasons of our marriage I was unaware of my behavior, and for other seasons I was aware, but didn't really want to change.

The questions of why we are the way we are and why we do what we do are complex. But even greater is the question of why we hang onto behavior that we know is unhealthy and hurtful. As I laid on my deathbed months earlier, I had very few regrets. However, my single greatest regret was my failure to honor Joanna through our married life.

Yes, I loved her, had been faithful to her, and knew that I would spend my life with her. She certainly had been all of that to me and more. However, as I lay motionless in ICU, I knew that I had not treated her as Christ would. I was sparse in my words of affirmation, clueless about some of her needs, careless about how I cared for her at her vulnerable moments, and generally took her for granted. I never said the words, but my basic attitude too often was, *She's a strong woman. She can take care of herself.*

I was right in my assessment. She usually did handle whatever neglect I gave, but I was horribly wrong in my approach. Obviously this was hardly the attitude a Christ-following husband should take.

My failure as a husband had the natural by-product that we rarely connected on a deeply spiritual level. Our prayer times together were infrequent and rarely had that sense of "flow" when two hearts are completely knitted. We rarely shared our spiritual experiences with each other. We really didn't know if it was safe to open up our souls and share deeply.

I also avoided conflict at all cost. I absolutely hated to argue with her. My avoidance of conflict often led to unhealthy patterns on my part. I became skilled at only giving her as much information as I wanted her to have so that I didn't have to deal with the potential conflict that might arise if she knew the full story. This wasn't a good foundation upon which to build a marriage.

I always had a little internal cringe whenever I performed a wedding ceremony and led the couple through their vows to love and to "cherish" one another. I had the nagging feeling that I barely knew what the word meant.

Our twenty seventh anniversary occurred while I was still in ICU. I knew that there was more reason for sadness than just my physical state. We were twenty seven years into our marriage and had raised three fantastic children together, but I knew that the years to come could be and must be better than the ones past. And I knew much of the responsibility for change had to be on my shoulders.

The foundation of our marriage had cracks. Rebuilding was possible. But, as with most processes of healthy change, it had to begin with an honest admission.

Through tears, I confessed to her that I had not honored her the way that I should have as a Christian husband. I had not treated her as Christ intended. I had failed her in many ways for many years. There was no way that I could recall all the times I had failed to honor her, but I could and did name a few specific examples of my failures.

Frankly, my timing was horrible and my approach was no better. Round One didn't go too well. Yet, I knew I was onto something. I knew she loved me enough to eventually forgive me. I knew I was dredging up hurtful things from our past—recent and distant—that were hard enough the first time around; now she had to live them again through my apology.

Sometimes it feels easier to "just not go there." We may not like the place we're in, but we can ignore it more easily if no one talks about it. I had to talk. I brought the subject up again. Each time I re-opened the wound and she felt the pain. To her credit, she was strong enough to walk through it. Healing gradually came.

It helped, I suppose, that neither of us had anywhere to go. She was my 24/7 caregiver through the majority of this healing process. It helped, as well, that I was flat-on-my-back humbled and needing her care. It helped that her spiritual gift of mercy was now released upon me as I had never experienced it before. It helped immensely that she loves God with all her heart and was determined to do what was right by our marriage, even if it wasn't easy.

Eventually, as my health improved, with our own house for sale and uncertain where we would live next, we met with a realtor to explore our options. The agent showed us a house that intrigued me. It was an old home with all the hardwood and character that Joanna loves. I inspected the property carefully and was impressed that for such an old home, it had an extremely solid foundation. The realtor explained that the house had actually been picked up, moved across town, and placed on a new foundation: Same house, new foundation.

In that house, I saw a picture of what God was doing in our marriage. As Joanna gradually believed my apology and my sincere desire to change, her heart opened to me more and more. The first layers of the new foundation were proving to be solid.

The layers that followed have come quite naturally. With my new resolve to honor her at all times:

- I have begun to live a lifestyle of full-disclosure, keeping nothing from her. Since my new value is to honor her—rather than avoid conflict or protect my image—I can freely admit bad decisions I have made in the past, insecurities I have, and feelings I am experiencing. As I open my heart to her, it is more natural for her to open her heart to me.

- I am allowing her into my soul journey. I'm eager for her input. I want to know her views. I value her wisdom and insight. I want her perspective on scripture. This is new territory for her, but with time she is freely entering in.

- I see her through new eyes. Rather than looking at her through the perspective of my own strengths or spiritual gifting, I see her for who God has made her to uniquely be. She is more caring, precious, and beautiful than I ever realized. How foolish I have been to miss the many nuances of her beauty through the years!

- I've become convinced that conflict isn't the thing to be most avoided. Worse than potential conflict is not dealing with issues that must be addressed. To my happy surprise, the more I am willing to face conflict, the less we seem to have. And, when we do have conflict, we're not operating from a base of fear. Fear always makes a miserable base. We're never at our best when we're responding out of fear. Love, it seems, is casting out fear (1 John 4:18).

Why are some couples strengthened by crisis and others destroyed by it?

We don't pretend to have some survival formula for every couple going through crises. However, we do want to testify that a couple with a marginal relationship can not only survive a crisis, but thrive in the midst of it.

One by-product of our new relationship is that Joanna and I seem to find reasons to laugh most every day. Recently, Joanna was out running errands and was gone longer than I expected. When she got back, I hugged her and said, "How can you light up my life if you don't darken my door?" I know, it sounds like a country song title, but she laughed and accepted my embrace.

We pray more, too. Now knitted together with stronger strands of trust and openness, our hearts more naturally open to God together.

I will still revert to old patterns from time to time. She'll still have a few layers of hurt to work through. But we both delight that the old house of our marriage has been placed on a new foundation. We always did like that old house. It's been around long enough to have plenty of character. It just needed a better base to stand on.

# REACTIONS

Shortly after returning from the road trip, I was given the privilege of sharing the story of my healing with the Salem Alliance Church family. Dr. Byrkit, my primary care physician who had given me the sermon in the hospital, approached me at the front of the church after I spoke and simply confirmed, "It's a miracle, not medicine."

However, upon hearing the news that I was now eating, my ENT doctor had a different reaction. I'm told that his first response was, "Who gave him permission to eat?!"

He wasn't happy. He was concerned. He had given me two guided tours of my inoperable throat. He had talked to the experts. He knew how severe my case was. He had reason for his worried reaction to my new daily activity.

His office called and requested that I set up an appointment. When I arrived, I was pleased to see that his speech/swallow therapist was there to meet me as well. She had worked with me with great diligence and special kindness, but with no real results.

I entered their office having already gained at least ten pounds. I was walking, talking, smiling and doing about everything with greater strength than when they had seen me two months earlier. Their concerns were quieted almost immediately as they observed me. I assured them that I would remain cautious as I re-entered the world of food and beverage, but I also assured them that I am confident God has me on a path of healing. The evidence of my progress was sitting before them.

The doctor seemed to breathe a sigh of relief as he admitted, "It's nothing short of a miracle. People don't just start swallowing."

By the end of summer, I only needed my feeding tube for hydration. I needed to show caution in what I attempted to eat and how fast I tried to eat it, but I was no longer dependent upon the tube for nutrition.

I didn't want to merely throw away our leftover cases of formula, but the company that sent it to me didn't take returns. Our former home health care nurse, Nora, offered to make a call for us to an agency that assists patients like me. Nora called and mentioned that I had leftover formula that I no longer needed.

The woman on the other end of the call knew of my original illness but hadn't heard any recent update of my condition. Upon hearing that the formula wasn't needed anymore, she became somber and fell silent.

Nora suddenly realized that she assumed I was dying or had already died.

"No. No! He's been healed! He's eating now!"

As Nora relayed the story to us, I was reminded of how blessed I am. My story could have turned out so very differently.

It was a joy to begin to get to share my story in various churches, including our home church. I found myself naturally telling pieces of my story in public places such as the barbershop during a haircut. I was aware, that as excited as I was about what God had done for me, there were some who would remain skeptical. In my frustration one night, I wrote this,

> I trust that this story will strengthen your faith. However, I understand that not everyone easily believes a story like this. I can't convince you of anything; all I can do is share my story and leave it for you to decide what to do with it. What I know for sure is that I didn't swallow for seventeen months and now I do. I believe God did this.
>
> You can come up with some other explanation if you want to. I can't stop you from it. But I'll just tell you that there's an unemployed spit cup in some dumpster in Southern Illinois. There's an empty yogurt container on the shelf by my desk that echoes a testimony to God's power. There's a pile of unused spit rags ready to

be thrown away instead of sitting next to a pillow. There's a forty-nine-year-old guy who is sleeping like he hasn't slept in eighteen months because he's no longer spitting the night through. There's now an additional seventeen pounds on his skinny frame. And, there is a turkey and cheese sandwich in hand as he prepares these words.

You can draw your own conclusion, but I am convinced that God did this.

# TAKING THE HEAT

It was only eight o'clock in the morning, but the temperature was already pushing 100 degrees as my daughter Anna and I stepped out of the car into the Mayo Clinic parking lot in Scottsdale, Arizona. Chimes greeted us by playing, "O What a Wonderful Feeling, O What a Beautiful Day." Evidently the clinic wanted us to think happy thoughts during our visit.

After months of attempting to get into Mayo, I was finally there. I was expectant. These doctors earned a great reputation for a reason. I accepted the fact that the doctors at OHSU never reached a diagnosis. No one would ever know what had about killed me. I'm content to leave that question in the mystery genre of my story.

However, my ongoing daily life gave evidence that something still hindered full recovery. I continued to have profound muscle weakness and odd skin coloration patterns. The diagnosis of Dermatomyositis that my local doctors gave never satisfied me. I wanted one more opinion, and I wanted it from the most respected source I could access.

Anna and Jeff lived in Scottsdale and proved to be very gracious hosts. Anna juggled her work in a university research lab so she could take me to my appointment. This required her to go into the lab at 4:15 in the morning to begin an experiment which she would finish later in the day, but she made no complaint.

We entered the clinic to be swept into a current of kindness and efficiency. Everyone was helpful. The staff seemed relaxed. They appeared to actually like working together. Kindness permeated each office. It appeared to me that Mayo had successfully staffed the clinic with a team of caring people. I felt valued.

My first appointment was with a doctor I was eager to see. He would be the one to oversee my case for the couple of days that I was to be there. Before I came, I learned that he has a reputation for being brilliant.

The clinic's atmosphere of friendliness suddenly changed as he entered the room. I quickly found him to be a man who viewed words as currency; he was the embodiment of "cheap." I surmised that he grew up in the Great Verbal Depression. Words are to be saved, not foolishly spent. His Rule of Operation—an unstated rule, obviously—was, "Never use a full sentence when a single word will do."

As I waited and watched, I found myself respecting him. His silence added to his aura of brilliance. Talking only delayed the opportunity for him to think. And as long as he was thinking about *me,* I wanted to give him all the time in the world. He shuffled through pages of my file, peered into the screen of his computer, and read medical reports on his phone. Occasionally he asked a clarifying question. I learned to make my answers concise.

When my appointment with him concluded, I was instructed to return to the scheduling desk. The receptionist there cautiously asked me how my time with the doctor went. Evidently he has a reputation for more than his brilliance.

"I thought he was great," I responded.

"Really? You mean he wasn't..." She stopped herself, choosing her words diplomatically. "Well, some patients just don't like him very well."

"I wasn't hoping to make a friend. I just want his medical help."

She breathed a sigh of relief, commended my approach, and explained the appointments with other specialists that were scheduled for me. I would see my doctor again when I completed the other exams.

I was instructed to undergo another Modified Barium Swallow test. Being a veteran of this simple procedure, I was relaxed as I was escorted into a bare hallway. Four small chairs were scattered along the wall facing a small TV. The Scottsdale Mayo had at least six beautiful waiting areas, but this wasn't one of them. The hard chairs lining the drab hall indicated that relatively few people have the need to find their way to this part of the building. It felt like the hall of shame.

A lone woman sat waiting. She made sure her back was turned to me as I took my seat. Instinctively, I knew what she was doing, even as she was attempting to hide from me. I sensed what she was feeling: awkward, embarrassed…ashamed.

I offered a simple hello but she kept her back turned to me.

Finally she spoke, "I'm not trying to be rude."

"I understand," I replied. "I have one, too."

"You do?" She asked with shocked surprise. She turned toward me, revealing a feeding tube into which she had been pouring formula.

I doubt that she had ever met anyone who shared her experience of having difficulty with swallowing. It's rare to meet someone in public who has a feeding tube inserted into their stomach. It's something we tend to hide and for her it seemed to bring with it shame.

I was not hungry, but I reached into my backpack, pulled out a leftover can of formula and a syringe and announced, "Let's have lunch together!"

She relaxed and smiled. The embarrassment and shame were gone. She began to talk freely. Her story spilled out faster than her formula. I had made a friend.

Her name was called too soon. She thanked me as she gathered her things and left for her exam. I never saw her again and regret that I didn't take the opportunity to tell her that Jesus seems to have a special heart for people who think they need to hide something. A woman—with far deeper reason for shame than my new friend—met Jesus at a well one noonday. To her great surprise, she encountered love where she anticipated rejection. In Jesus she found acceptance, grace, and hope. I wish I could have told my new friend that the God of the Bible is surprisingly a God who understands pain and rejection, suffering and shame, scars and crosses. He's loving enough to handle whatever we're hiding under our "shirt."

My days at Mayo became a flurry of filling out forms, phlebotomy (nineteen vials of blood), and fascinating conversations with friendly doctors. The days concluded with a final visit with my initial doctor—Dr. Sparse Words. He had already gathered the results from my other appointments.

As he finished reviewing my records, he turned toward me to tell me his conclusion. This was the entire reason for which I traveled all the way to Arizona. Significant money and time led me to this moment. This was the only reason I was here: to hear this doctor's verdict. I leaned forward in my chair to hear the news.

Peering over his glasses, he looked me in the eye and announced,

"Mee-ster Stoom-bo, I can say with cer-tain-ty, you have Der-mat-o-my-o-si-tis."

He spoke in staccato, every syllable clearly emphasized. He also had a great accent, the type of which made him seem even more brilliant.

My spirit sank as I heard the words. This was the diagnosis I had been treated for over the last year. He made no claims that this was what nearly killed me at first; he was simply diagnosing what was going on now in my body.

As I sat before him, I couldn't help but feel disappointed. This wasn't the news I wanted. What I had hoped to hear was, "Mr. Stumbo, they've misdiagnosed your disease. We have a remedy that will get you back to normal in no time."

I gathered my thoughts, and asked him what I could expect for the future.

He was thoughtful in his response, "Vill you e-ver run an ultra-mar-a-thon a-gain? No."

A second doctor that I'd already seen joined us, added his agreement about the diagnosis and concluded, "You have a condition that you will have to learn to live with."

I was sobered.

The doctors verified that the IVIG treatment I receive is appropriate. They recommend that I immediately stop taking the oral medication I was prescribed. I was eager to do this because I had always questioned why I was on it. They explained that the medication, rather than helping me, may have been contributing to my anemic condition.

I left Mayo grateful for their thoroughness and kindness, but in a daze. In the days that followed, I tried to gather my thoughts and capture my conclusions in a few statements:

- I believe that it is good to be told the truth and accept it. This is my condition. I need to face it. I respect those who face the truth about themselves, and I want to be one of those people.

- I believe that this is all the more reason to continue to pray for healing. If God continues to heal me completely, the statements from these doctors will only add to the glory God receives for the healing.

- I need to accept that without divine intervention, medicine will only be able to do so much for me. According to the National Association of Neurological Disorders, "There is no cure for Dermatomyositis." That's pretty straightforward. A few months ago I wrote that I was seeking to: "Accept today. Battle for a better tomorrow." In my post-Mayo reflection, I realize that this is more appropriate than ever.

Eventually I add a fourth summary response,

- Ultimately, the grand story is not about what I can or can't do—it is about what God is doing. And, God is working for His glory.

# DIAGNOSED BUT NOT DEFINED

I now carry a label. I have a diagnosis. It has a name. There's not a great deal known about it, but it is in the annals of medical knowledge.

I'm not happy about my diagnosis. But it's the reality of my situation. And, I fully recognize, it is a reality for an increasing percentage of the population. It seems like most people have one diagnosis or another these days.

In the words of others much more intelligent than me, "How then shall we live?"

I don't pretend to have the final answer on this matter. I merely admit that I, as a novice to the subject, am bothered by much of what I hear people say. Our language betrays our beliefs. When we really listen to our own words, we often realize that they reveal the true convictions of our hearts.

On this matter of having received a medical diagnosis, I hear many people say things like,

"I have cancer."

"I have _____."

Sometimes, people personalize the statement even further by saying,

"I am a diabetic."

"I am a _____."

I understand why we speak this way. Our western approach to medicine certainly embeds this language deeper into us. However, oddball or renegade that I am, I have a problem with this language, especially for all those who claim to be followers of Jesus. Allow me to explain my current view.

First, speaking in such ways reveals that we view ourselves first and foremost as physical beings. We think of ourselves primarily from the standpoint of our physical bodies. We get this view from western medicine. Countless magazines and media reaffirm it. The time we spend in front of a mirror affirms it as well. To some degree we may be aware that we also have a soul and spirit, but evidently these aspects of the human person are secondary to our fundamental understanding of who we are. Through the worldview of western culture, we are primarily physical beings.

Allow me to make the happy announcement that we are far more than a physical body! When we see our bodies as the temporary residence for our eternal soul, our perspective starts to shift. When we accept that the real us—the part of us that makes us us—cannot be pricked with a needle or studied under a scan, our paradigm changes.

As a Christ-follower, I have the hope and confidence that when my physical body expires, my finest life is actually just beginning. My soul and spirit live on. Like a tenant, I dwell in a body for this era of my existence, but my life isn't dependent on it. Someday we will be given resurrection bodies like that of Jesus, but who we are—our true personhood—lives whether our body does or not.

Currently, my own physical body has not been one hundred percent restored, but my soul is in better shape than it has ever been. In other words, because we are more than physical beings, we can be alive in spirit while dying in body. Our souls can flourish even as our bodies diminish. Have you not seen this phenomenon in some aging saints? They may shuffle along with an unsteady step, but when you look them in the eye or listen to their words, it is obvious that they are vibrant in spirit.

Let's not allow ourselves to be defined by our bodies.

Second, let's not be defined by our diagnosis. Our illness—whatever label it has been given—is not us. It does not describe who we really are. It should not become our identity. The doctors have declared to me, "You have Dermatomyositis." That is my diagnosis. But instead, I prefer to declare, "I have Jesus."

I'm not denying my diagnosis. I'm just determined to not let it define me. I don't intend to scold anyone and I fully understand how embedded it is into our language and culture, but I'm bothered when I hear people say statements such as "I'm a diabetic."

I don't like that language because I don't want our identity to be summarized by our illness. Your physical body may well indeed be afflicted with diabetes, but it's not *who* you are. Diabetes is a real and difficult issue. I sympathize with those who suffer from it.

But to my Christ-following friends, I ask, "Wouldn't it be better to remind ourselves of who we really are?"

I challenge you to study the scripture for yourself and add to the following list. The New Testament proclaims followers of Christ to be:

Blessed with every spiritual blessing (Ephesians 1:3)
Chosen before the creation of the world (Ephesians 1:4)
Adopted into His family (Ephesians 1:5)
Redeemed through His blood (Ephesians 1:7)
Sealed with the Holy Spirit (Ephesians 1:13)
Seated with Christ in heavenly places (Ephesians 2:6)
Saved by His grace (Ephesians 2:8)
God's unique workmanship (Ephesians 2:10)
A dwelling place of the Holy Spirit (Ephesians 2:22)

Third, I challenge you to believe with me that our present situation is not our permanent situation. God is not done working in us. He is the God who is always at work on behalf of His children. Please have confidence with me that He will change our situation or change our response to our situation. He will either rescue us from our crisis or renew us in it. Whatever our situation, whatever our outcome, we know with certainty that we are not stuck, trapped, or abandoned. He may come in surprising ways. He may come at unexpected times. But of this we can be sure: He does come.

Allow me to say it again. As long as we have God, we have hope. And I joyfully celebrate with you that we will *always* have God.

Finally, please believe with me that our doctor's prognosis is not prophetic. My doctor at Mayo said I'd never do certain things I once did. He's smart. But he doesn't get to have the final say. Someone of Higher Authority does. Jesus gets to have the final say. We have plenty of good physicians here on earth. But we have the Great Physician in heaven.

# UP IN THE AIR

"Pakistan? Really?"

I could see the concern on people's faces as they heard the news. I was hardly the picture of health. Was it wise for me to travel halfway around the globe?

Three years earlier a small team of Christian doctors, Bible translators, Christian educators, and other "international workers" in Pakistan had invited me to speak at their annual conference. Rather than giving the assignment to someone else as I was near death or during my long era of recovery, they held the spot open for me. And, they prayed.

I appreciated their faith. I appreciated the commitment that they made every day of their lives to serve Jesus Christ in a land that is ninety-eight percent Islamic. I was honored by their desire to have me bring God's Word to them.

They didn't pressure me. The conference leadership team gave me complete freedom to not fulfill the commitment. I was hesitant to say a final yes. However, when it was suggested that I could bring a caregiver along with me, I seized the idea. My son, Josiah, had proven to be a great caregiver. He was now a college graduate and had a job that was flexible enough to allow this kind of travel. His own intrigue about serving Jesus internationally would only be enhanced by such a trip. And I coveted the opportunity to spend some extended time with one of my sons.

I rarely used my feeding tube anymore as my ability to swallow continued to strengthen. However, under the advisement of my doctor, I left it in just in case I had some reversal of my health status as I traveled. He didn't want me to risk the possibility of dehydration.

My greater concern was whether my muscles, which tend to complain loudly after being stuck in the same position, could handle the fifteen hour flight from San Francisco to Dubai. A few shorter flights were involved as well to ultimately connect us from Portland to Islamabad, but I had less reason to be concerned about these.

The marathon flight took us over the North Pole and then over cities I couldn't pronounce. As the hours passed, I noticed that the attendants of this Emirates Air were hardworking and amazingly able to keep a good attitude in spite of being trapped inside the same metal tube as the rest of us for these long hours.

Late in the flight, I walked to the rear of the plane to use the bathroom. A short line had formed and I tried to find a place to stay out of traffic. I found myself in the corner of the galley as a half-dozen flight attendants from as many nationalities busily completed their tasks. Their hard work, cooperation with each other, and professionalism impressed me.

As one attendant passed me I commented, "You guys are amazing! You've been at this for over fourteen hours and you're still going at it. Thanks for taking such good care of us."

My comment stopped the attendant in her tracks. She looked me in the eye carefully and repeated back to me what I had just said, "You mean you think we did a good job taking care of you?"

I could tell that she didn't know if she should take me seriously or not. Other attendants stopped their work to listen to our brief exchange.

"Yes," I repeated. "I think you've done a great job, especially for how long this flight is. Thank you!"

"This is very rare," she said in a somber, but appreciative manner. "We don't hear that kind of comment very often."

When I arrived in Pakistan, I shared this brief conversation with one of the international workers. He explained, "Gratitude is probably lacking in many cultures, but in this culture it is especially rare. Local theology requires people to do acts of kindness to earn favor with God. So if, for example, a beggar asks you for money and you give it to him, he will not thank you for he is the one who has done *you* a favor."

"Really?" I was surprised by his answer and wanted to know more.

"Yes. In fact, rather than thanking you, the beggar is likely to ask you for another gift so that you can have another opportunity to do good."

Immediately I could see how gratitude is not fostered by such a worldview. At least in America we make an attempt at valuing gratitude with our celebration of Thanksgiving. We may not practice it well on that day or throughout the year, but it is understood as a value.

Soon, however, the tables would be turned and I would see how weak our American Christian theology is in other areas.

One day during the conference, the international workers had a training seminar on how to handle crises. The list of subjects presented was unlike any seminar list I had ever seen:

- What to do in an attempted carjacking
- How to react when a hand grenade is thrown in your vicinity
- How to react to a possible suicide bombing
- Safety tips for avoiding abduction

On the list went. I observed the seminar with mild curiosity at first. Yet, soon I realized that for every scenario presented, someone in the room had a first-person or one-person-removed story to match.

I sat humbled. I had privately prided myself in my willingness to travel for a few days of ministry with a feeding tube still attached to my stomach. Meanwhile, most of these saints have given decades of their lives to serve in regions most of us would never visit for a day. Unknown to any of us in the room at the time—or virtually anyone in the world for that matter—a number of these Christian workers were serving in the same town from which Osama Bin Laden would later be abducted. While they ministered the love of Jesus through their hospital, just on the other side of town the world's most-wanted terrorist carried on his clandestine work.

The willingness of this team to serve, even after surviving threats, grenades, and bombings, stood to me in stark contrast to so much of American Christianity. The visible fruit from their labors, sowing in such hard soil, is limited. The "thanks" that they receive is minimal. The "perks" are almost nonexistent. The danger, omnipresent.

Yet, year after dry year they serve, believing that ultimately their labor is not in vain in the Lord (1 Corinthians 15:58).

I've stated that their service stands in contrast to much of American Christianity. Allow me to be more specific. Much American theology seems to be based on two powerful American "values": *rapidity* and *ease*. As many others have observed, whether it is the service we receive at a store, the food we eat, or even our faith, we are a society enamored with the quick and easy.

I speak for myself as well. I am very American in these matters. I am a product of an American version of Christian theology. Recognizing this causes me to ask myself two questions. Maybe you ask these questions along with me.

First, do I assume that if God doesn't answer a prayer the *moment* I want Him to, that He has said no to me?

This question probes at my American need to have everything *now*. Waiting isn't on our list of highly cherished values. It is common for us to reach the conclusion that if we don't receive an immediate answer to prayer, we doubt that He'll ever answer it. We can easily adopt an "I tried and it didn't work" attitude.

I've often gathered with a team of elders, as instructed in James 5, to anoint a sick person with oil and pray for them. If God doesn't heal the person instantly, there can be a sense of disappointment. We can too quickly conclude that God has said no.

But isn't it possible that God *is* going to do something miraculous in the person, but has a timetable of His own? Isn't it possible that God is doing something miraculous in that person right at that very moment, but we just don't have eyes to see it yet? Just because God doesn't show up in an evident way the moment we ask, doesn't necessarily mean that He's not working.

I confess that there have been times in my life where I've treated prayer as if it has an expiration date.

*Well, we prayed for that yesterday and I don't see any difference today. I guess that prayer didn't go anywhere.*

Conversely, is it possible that our prayers are remembered in heaven long after we've forgotten them on earth? Is it possible that when a prayer of faith rises to the throne of God, it lingers before Him like incense? (See Revelation 8:3-5.)

If I have learned anything from this mysterious journey that I've been on, it is that God does things in His own timing. The scriptures repeatedly instruct us to "wait" on Him. (See Psalm 27:14 for starters.) The scriptures are clear that God sees time from a different viewpoint than we do. (Check out 2 Peter 3:8-9.) Many of the greatest stories of scripture have a long waiting period in them. David's story in 1 Samuel is evidence of this. He's anointed as the next King of Israel in chapter sixteen, but fifteen chapters later he's still not on the throne.

Or, turn to the account of Zechariah and Elizabeth in Luke 1. It's more than a good Christmas story. The parents of John the Baptist have lived a lifetime of unanswered prayer. For decades—for the vast majority of their lives—they are childless. Zechariah is a priest. They are a righteous couple. They are God's chosen people. Evidently, godliness doesn't exempt us from disappointment.

One day, Zechariah is chosen to enter the temple to offer incense before the Lord. He is alone in this holy place. Or so he assumes. Suddenly, he freezes in fear. He's not alone. An angel is speaking to him, "Your prayer has been heard."

A son is promised. A very special son. A Spirit-filled son. The forerunner for the Messiah.

Zechariah responds with skepticism, "How can I be sure of this? I'm old and my wife is getting up there in years, too."

In case you think that his answer is a mere question of curiosity or a factual question to gain a little more information, the angel's response indicates something different.

"I am Gabriel. I stand in the presence of God! I have been sent to speak to you. I was sent to tell you good news. But because you didn't believe me, you aren't going to be able to say another word until what I have spoken comes to pass. And, it will come true in its proper time!"

Evidently, the good angel Gabriel didn't appreciate leaving the throne of God and crossing into our world, only to have an aging human doubt him.

I hear in Zechariah's answer the voice of one who has lost hope for this answer to prayer long ago. He, no doubt, prayed in faith during one season of his life. But time had worn him down. He was no longer expectant, hopeful, or waiting.

You might read the story differently, but I don't believe Zechariah had prayed for a child on that day inside the temple. His answer to the angel gives no indication that he was still praying for this anymore at all. When Gabriel announces, "Your prayer has been heard," I assume that he is referring to Zechariah's prayer from years past. This isn't an answer to a current prayer but an old prayer.

We serve a God who answers old prayers. Since God views time differently than we do, and since His plans are far different than we can fathom, He's not bound by human time frames. He can do things in an instant if He so desires. But sometimes His plan more beautifully unfolds over a lifetime...or even over centuries.

Let me say it plainly. You will become discouraged in your relationship with God if you insist that He operate on your schedule. Many people have walked away from faith because—from their vantage point—God didn't come through for them when they thought He should. Many a person has missed a miracle in their finances, relationships, body, or soul because they assumed that because they didn't see any evidence of His work that He wasn't doing anything. The American need for immediate results has shipwrecked the faith of many.

Faith can't be microwaved. God's not confined to man-made deadlines. Any teachings or perspectives on faith that ignore this are unhelpful, and quite likely even dangerous.

I see myself in Zechariah. Maybe you do as well.

# GETTING OFF EASY

The second question I must ask myself—being the product of American theology that I am—is: Do I assume that if God doesn't answer a prayer in the *manner* I want Him to that He has abandoned me?

This question probes at my American need to have everything *easy*. Suffering isn't on our list of highly cherished values. Suffering, in our minds, is even worse than waiting. Now, in all fairness, I don't know that suffering is desirable in any culture. I'm not saying we should desire it. But, some cultures have certainly understood far better than Americans that suffering is normal and beneficial. Let me say it again, some see suffering as a natural part of living on this planet and an effective tool God uses.

I think the Apostle Peter would have been one of those who viewed life this way. He wrote, "Dear friends, do not be surprised at the painful trial you are suffering, as though something strange were happening to you" (1 Peter 4:12).

Meanwhile, some strands of American theology teach that God would never use such harsh methods as physical illness in our lives. Their teaching leaves the impression that if something goes poorly in our lives or bodies, something must be wrong with us. It is immediately assumed that sin is present, Satan is winning, or faith is absent.

I acknowledge that all of these options are possible. We may need to repent of sin. We must resist and rebuke the devil. We could always benefit from an enlargement of our faith. But, I also believe that a fourth option is possible: a God of love is reshaping our lives.

I've asked audiences, "What takes more faith? To believe God for healing or to keep believing in God when no healing comes? To cling to God for a miracle or to still cling to God when no miracle is in sight?"

Much of American theology celebrates the Christ of healing but doesn't know what to do with the Christ of suffering. We honor Christ our Healer, and honor Him we should! We should also honor Christ our Sufferer.

Looking back, I realize that God could have healed me at any time and in any manner He chose. I would have loved for Him to have done it a year earlier, in a public setting with more dramatic effect. I would have loved to have gone from zero to one hundred percent swallowing in ten seconds. He could have done this if He had so desired. Yet, He chose a longer, sequestered, and more subtle route.

Meanwhile, I can't answer the question as to why He healed my swallow, but not some of my other muscles' issues, allowing me to run again. Will I ever run long distances again? I have no way of knowing that right now. Will I ever live a pain free day of life on earth? I'm not sure. But I am convinced and happily testify that He's not done working...neither in my life nor yours.

I know that many people have an "I don't know what God is doing in my life" story. I know that readers of this book represent countless "unanswered" prayers, or to say it better, prayers that we have yet to see answered in the manner that we desire.

I also know from personal experience that when healing doesn't come quickly, destructive forces can find their way into our hearts. When the healing of our situation—be it financial, relational, emotional, physical, or spiritual—doesn't come quickly:

- Disappointment with God can set in.
- Discouragement can pull us down.
- Despair lurks in the shadows.
- Ugly attitudes such as jealousy, envy, and anger threaten to spread like mold in our hearts.

This list of potential downfalls is much longer. There is good reason that the saints through the ages have referred to the "dark night of the soul."

And, it seems that there are demons waiting for us in those dark corridors. They prey upon us at those times. Whether they are involved in the illness or problem or not, I don't know. But what I do know is that they seek to capitalize on it. They seize the season of our crisis as an opportunity to shoot their arrows at us.

From my understanding of scripture and life, the demons' primary attack is upon our thoughts. The primary battleground is in our heads. Their frequently used tool is the power of a lie. Lies that are suggested to our minds must be identified and resisted.

Satan, the father of lies (John 8:44), and his minions seem to have a few that are particularly successful during times of crisis:

- God doesn't really love you.
- If God was really good, this wouldn't be happening to you right now.
- Maybe God cares about other people. Maybe God will answer their prayers. But not you. You don't count. You don't matter to Him.

The list of lies is much longer. It is vital for us to identify them as they enter our thoughts. There is good reason that the scriptures instruct us to "take up the shield of faith, with which you can extinguish all the flaming arrows of the evil one" (Ephesians 6:16). We don't have to receive or believe the lies that come to us. But, it is a genuine battle.

A friend of mine, Dr. Frank Chan, teaches, "Lies born in these times of pain are powerful. The presence of pain makes the lie feel true."

Great spiritual progress can be made as we identify the lies bouncing around in our own heads, and replace them with the truth of what God says about us.

One truth is that while God seems hidden or silent, He is still at work. I can't tell you exactly what God is doing in your life right now, but I can tell you the kinds of things that He is known to do in the midst of His silence. When your prayer isn't being answered in the timing or manner that you desire, there are numerous possibilities for what may well be happening in the meantime:

- Your faith is being refined (1 Peter 1:3-7).

- Your maturity is being deepened (Hebrews 5:7-9).
- Your character is being shaped and a harvest prepared (Hebrews 12:4-11).
- Your view of God is being enlarged (Job 38-42).
- Your testimony is becoming known. Angels, demons, saints, and sinners alike watch and take notice, "Look! She is hanging onto God even though He's not coming through for her as she'd like." "Look! He still loves God, even though God is completely confusing him right now" (Ephesians 3:10).
- Finally, I want to testify, when healing doesn't come quickly, God is working and He's working for His glory! The Potter's hands are still damp, the wheel is still spinning, the clay is still being formed. He's not done. The Master Artist still has some work to do (Isaiah 64:8).

Years ago I was on a pleasant jog through a wooded trail. The trail remains one of my favorites. Miles of trees, ponds, blackberries, birds, and abandoned fields surrounded me. As I made my way through the woods and weeds, I began to complain to God about a particular situation I was facing. Looking back, I can't even remember what the issue was. But, at the time, it seemed like a big enough problem to be disturbed over and to whine to God about.

After a few twists and turns of the trail, I felt like I heard God deliver a message to my spirit, "What if I'm working on more than your personal happiness right now?"

"What? You mean there is something bigger than my personal happiness?"

He didn't answer. He didn't need to answer. I had, in a moment's time, been granted a higher perspective. I realized that I was evaluating my circumstances through the lens of how much they benefited me. If my circumstances made me happy, God was good. If my circumstances didn't make me happy my response was, "God, where are you? What's going on? Don't you see what's going on here?"

And God, in His kindness, lifted my view. It only took a couple minutes for my perspective to get a "faith lift" on my favorite trail that day. However, on this difficult marathon of my health challenges, it has taken a couple years to gain the perspective I've just shared with you.

Please understand this. Some teaching may be great teaching; it just may not be the right time for you to receive it. Perhaps today you are in such pain you can't receive all I've shared in these pages. That's okay. I wouldn't have been able to receive all of them at various points of my trial. Leave them for a later day. For this moment, simply know that God travels this trail with you. He may be distant and silent, but He is there. Replace the lies of Satan with the truth of scripture, "Never will I leave you; never will I forsake you" (Hebrews 13:5 and Deuteronomy 31:6).

I doubt if He would have bothered to tell us this if we wouldn't have reason to question it at times. The challenge that comes to us is: Will we believe our feelings or believe the scripture? It is a difficult challenge. I didn't rise to meet it every day as I should have. But at the two year point in this journey I can testify that, yes, He has been there all along.

# THE DUBAI DJ

I gained much from my time in Pakistan. Josiah's worldview was enlarged as well. It had been a great trip and my health seemed no worse for the travels. With deep respect in our hearts for the team of workers there, we left to return to the United States by way of Dubai—a fascinating city in the desert, complete with an indoor snow ski hill.

I don't know if it was the Spirit's prompting or that my adventuresome spirit had already been maxed out by ten days of international travel, but as our team headed out to explore the Persian Gulf, I opted to stay by our hotel. After taking a few pictures of the neighborhood mosque, I found my way back to the hotel and took the elevator to the health club on the twelfth floor.

Exercising isn't what it once was for me. I once loved the feel of my heart pumping, lungs billowing, and sweat pouring. Four or five times a week, I would happily challenge myself to another round of laps, weights, or some form of conditioning. It was a challenge. It was a joy. Its fruits were easily seen. Those days are now just a memory.

I attempted to begin my "workout" this day in the same manner I always did in my prime—seated on a large exercise ball to do a few stomach and back routines to ease my way into the event. This day, however, I had little motivation to attempt what little I could still do.

I sat on the ball, mildly stretching some angry ligaments and muscles. I hoped that if I sat there long enough, some mysterious motivation would arrive. Pain—aggravating and nagging, but not debilitating—accompanied virtually every movement and dared motivation to enter the room. As I attempted to stretch, my mind drifted to the fallen state in which I found myself: my body a shell of what it once was, my future uncertain, my spirit low.

My mind wandered to the coming weekend's resignation. I was returning home to announce to the five services of Salem Alliance Church that our rich and mysterious eight year journey there was coming to an end.

A year after stepping down from my role as lead pastor, I was now convinced that it was time to resign from my part-time associate role and step aside completely. The church was being led well. Joanna and I had a definite sense in our hearts of being released from our call to the church. The work of the ministry is never completed on this earth, but sometimes our role in a specific ministry is.

The coming resignation seemed to climax the last few years of my life—years that had been marked by unanswered questions. As I sat, stretched, and stalled any real form of exercise, my own thoughts mocked me.

*I had numerous invitations to serve other places the few years before I became ill. Some of them were great opportunities! Maybe I've been a fool for the decisions I made to stay where I was. Would I have even become ill if I had taken one of those offers? Would my life be better now? I thought I was doing the right thing at the time, but maybe I was a fool.*

Slowly my depressing thoughts were interrupted. I gradually became aware of a song quietly playing on the health club sound system. When I first walked in the room I was aware that gentle music was playing—a collection of simple piano solos I didn't recognize. It became nothing more than pleasant background noise driving away complete silence.

Unthinking, my spirit began to sing along, "He leadeth me, He leadeth me."

*No,* my mind responded, *I'm in a health club on top of a hotel in the United Arab Emirates. I can't be hearing a Christian hymn right now.*

Yet, undeniably the song beautifully continued,

"He leadeth me. He leadeth me. By His own hand He leadeth me."

*God, help me always believe just that.*

Still sitting on the exercise ball, I began to cry softly. I mouthed the words as two full verses and choruses of the old hymn played on.

"His faithful follower I would be.
For by His hand He leadeth me."

Encouragement arrived as I realized, *What are the odds that this song would be playing in this place at this exact time?*

*Yes, Lord, you are leading me. I believe this. I trust you for this. Forgive me for being so fearful at times. Thank you for being so kind as to deliver a hymn to my wrestling heart.*

I was the only person in the club, but I was far from alone. I bowed my head and quietly prayed, "If you became a DJ in a Dubai hotel for me today, I think I can trust you to select the songs that compose my life. Keep leading, Lord. I'll try to keep following."

# PACKIN' ONE LESS THING

I returned from the international trip grateful for the experience, and grateful I was given the strength to complete it. I dreaded giving my resignation at church in all five services, but saw the value in communicating the message personally to as many people as possible. If I had to say good-bye, I would at least try to say it well.

Making the resignation easier was the fact that in God's kind timing, He had graciously provided an interim pastoral position for us at Fox Island Alliance Church, two hundred miles north in Washington. I would be able to work full-time again which was important to me for two reasons. First, the income we were receiving from our disability insurance was coming to an end. Within days of receiving our final payment from the insurance company, my interim employment began. God's financial provision couldn't have been more obvious. Second, I felt that an interim role was perfect for me as a testing ground for my health status. If my body was ready to work again full-time, I would be grateful. If my body couldn't handle it, at least I would only have a short-term commitment.

Meanwhile, I was about to cross the milestone of my fiftieth birthday. I received my best present early. It wasn't something someone gave me. It was something which was taken from me. A guy should be grateful for whatever tools and resources are used to spare and sustain his life, but that doesn't mean he can't be glad to see them go.

In the midst of a very full week of good-byes, closure, packing, celebrations, sermon preparation, and generally trying to wrap things up in my final days at the church, I slipped over to the local hospital and walked out minutes later feeding-tube-less. I was almost giddy with joy. For the first time in almost two years, I had nothing attached to my body. No tubes, machines, monitors, PICC lines, IVs, wound vacuums, or anything! I was attachment free and I was grateful.

# FOOL

It's Saturday night. We've made our move to Washington. I'm now an interim pastor. I open the double doors of the church sanctuary and find the light switch panel. Once the doors close behind me, the fan of a hidden furnace is the only sound I hear. I am alone. I've spent many Saturday nights in a place like this. Tonight I will walk the pews...for tomorrow I will stand in the pulpit.

Once again I've agreed to stand before a church congregation and tell my story of the last two years. I know why people want to hear it. People like stories of crisis, healing, God's intervention, and hope. More significantly, these embracing and loving people care about us, have prayed for us, and want to know more of the story than the little pieces of it they've heard off and on through the months.

I've told the story many times now to groups small and large. I know what lines will make people laugh. I know which lines will be hard for me to repeat. I know my story and I know it's not going to be easy to tell it again.

For the last few months I've been able to avoid having very many conversations about my health. I've been able to settle in to a new norm and go about daily life without a continual focus on medical issues. Pain awaits me as I awake in the morning if it hasn't already been awakening me in the night. My muscles still quarrel with me throughout the day. I'm grateful that none of the pain is debilitating. My quality of life has drastically improved even in recent months. Yet, the simplest task of getting out of a chair or pouring a glass of juice still bring reminders that discomfort and exertion are virtually omnipresent these days.

Omnipresent, but not omnipotent—they don't hold ultimate power. The ultimate power, the final say, resides in my soul and spirit. How I respond, the attitudes I choose, the metaphors I accept, the posture of dependence upon the Holy Spirit...these wield final say and greater authority than nagging nerves and melancholy muscles.

I've been learning to accept the level of activity I can participate in and not be too distraught by those things I can't do at this time. The people around me seem to have accepted it as well. Life has found a new post-crisis normalcy. I don't love the new norm, but it's certainly livable. Daily life has gone from barely tolerable to manageable...and some days, even pleasant.

But tonight, as I pray through the church sanctuary, I'm reminded again of the whole journey...the trails I once ran, the church I once led, the sudden reversal of my health, the days of teetering between life and death, the hallucinations—humorous and horrendous—the first signs of healing followed by long months of little progress, the seventeen months of living without eating, the continuous need to spit, the frustration of a clogged feeding tube, the desperate prayers in our rental car, the utter shock of eating the first bites of yogurt, the joy of re-entering community and ministry, the hope that perhaps tomorrow will be better than today...and emotionally I don't really want to face it all again. It's hard to put myself back into those memories and allow another congregation of people entrance into my heart.

My state, it seems, has not gone unnoticed. It's as if Satan stands in the background mocking me. I thought I could hear his hot whispers all week, but now the voice comes with all its infiltrating power.

"Fool!" he hisses. "You're going to stand up there again and tell a bunch of people that God is good. Well, if He's so good, why did any of this happen in the first place? Remember the life you once had? Look at what's been taken from you! Who were you serving the whole time this all took place? Some God you serve! Look where it's gotten you!"

I sigh. His lies always have slices of truth in them.

"Oh, shut up," I eventually groan.

My response doesn't strike me as sounding very spiritual, but tonight it's sufficient to keep the upper hand. Despair will not win this time. I've been down this path on worse nights than this. I've fought this battle already. I've claimed Peter's words from John 6 as my own, "Where else can I turn? Jesus, you alone have the words of eternal life."

I've considered my options and have reached my conclusion with Job, "Though he slay me, yet will I trust him."

With the assaulted Martin Luther I declare, "I cannot recant. Here I stand. I can do no other."

Yes, I will declare again the goodness of God.

Satan sulks away and I take the offensive. Every pew is prayed over and declarations fill the room:

"Greater is He that is in us than the one who fights against us. Greater is He that wants to forgive, heal, restore, and bless than he who wants to rob, discourage, and destroy. I celebrate that this place is dedicated for purposes of God. This church was established for the praise and glory of Jesus. Tomorrow, in this place, we're once again going to do what this church was made for. May praise fill this place. May salvation come to this place. May healing arise in this place. I declare that this is a place where Christ is found, discouragement is defeated, sin is abandoned, and grace is discovered."

I reach the front row and then the platform. I rest for a moment on the piano bench and begin to pick out the chords of an old hymn with my right hand.

*I need thee,*
*O I need thee.*
*Every hour I need thee.*
*O bless me now my Savior,*
*I come to thee.*

Yes, I will stand behind the pulpit again. I will tell my story again. I will once again declare my convictions and conclusions:

"God is good and can only be good. You may not like your current life circumstances, I haven't always liked mine. But He's the God of the light and the darkness. Too much American theology implies that He is the God of the good times only. He's bigger than that. Hang on to Him. Trust Him. He hasn't lost hold of you. If your own faith has been too battered, hang onto someone else's faith. Someone is believing for you."

# MORE CHAPTERS TO BE WRITTEN

In the opening words of this book I acknowledged that I stalled the writing of it. Once I finally got started, the writing of the story has gone as well as I could hope for a rookie author. Six months have now passed and the words I first penned have come back to me dozens of times, "To write a story is to experience it again. A story must be relived to be recorded."

I've found the "reliving" to be a healthy process. I trust you have benefited from reading this account. I know I'm the better for having recorded it.

As I bring this account to a close, I have an assurance that more chapters of my life are still to be written. And, I have reason to believe I can say the same for you. Your story and mine are part of a grand narrative, the eternal story of the God of All Creation at work in the lives of the people He created. God's not done writing yet. Neither are we. How amazing that we are co-authors with God in the story of life.

I've written many of the final chapters of this book from a small cottage in upstate New York. I'm here for the week as the evening speaker at the Delta Lake Family Bible Conference. The kind people here are a delight to be with and preach to. This is my third trip here in the last seven years. I happily accepted the invitation to return knowing that I'd be refreshed by my time here and that I'd have time during the day to write.

I've not been disappointed. It's been a rich week and I find myself now writing the final chapter to this edition of my story.

I type these words as ninety yards away a small group of runners are completing the annual "Simpson Circle Challenge." The Simpson Circle is a road—just a hair under a quarter mile in length by my calculation—that functions as the heart of the conference grounds. Inside the circle are park benches and a pleasant gazebo, a large lawn just perfect for Frisbee or a water fight, and the historic tabernacle—the thousand seat meeting place for our nightly gatherings of worship. On the perimeter of the circle are cottages where gracious people stay for a week or an entire summer. Front porches with lawn or rocking chairs welcome all who pass. Smiles are as abundant as the ice cream shakes at night.

The "Simpson Circle Challenge" is an annual fundraiser. The conference center is greatly assisted by their summer staff, a couple dozen of whom are college bound when summer ends. The "Challenge" raises scholarship funds for these staff members. I've enjoyed participating in the event when I come here and find satisfaction in helping the next generation fund their college education. Not everyone would consider four hours of running around a circle a great way to spend the afternoon, but I always loved the camaraderie of the event and the cause it supported.

Three years ago, when I was here last, I broke the "Simpson Circle Challenge" record. Yes, they do keep records of such things around here. It was a fun day of running as I logged 132 laps (about thirty two miles.) I felt strong. I felt happy. I couldn't have imagined that it was one of the last long runs I would ever complete.

I'm walking strong now and, on some days, I attempt to "run" a few hundred yards. My stride isn't natural yet, but I'm not giving up. Most days, however, it doesn't feel wise to even try. My body sends out various warning flares that I'm not ready to run yet.

I find God's timing interesting that as I type these very words, my former running companions are carrying on the tradition. As I close my story about this "marathon" that I've run the past thirty two months, the race I once won goes on outside my door.

True to their pattern of graciousness, they invited me to walk the first lap with them today. I showed up at the starting line with a measure of awkwardness. I felt honored to be present, but I was keenly aware that I'm no longer the man I was the last time I stood in this place.

As the leader of the event gave final instructions to the runners, he made an announcement:

"From this day forward the Simpson Circle Challenge will be renamed the John Stumbo Annual Challenge." I'm rarely speechless. But at this moment I didn't know how to respond. I hung my head, fearful that I seemed unappreciative, yet truly not knowing what to say.

*Did he really just say what I think I heard him say? I didn't see that coming.*

Without delay, a prayer is prayed, the countdown given, and we're off for Lap One. Like the pace car at a NASCAR race, I walk the first lap with the cheerful participants in stride behind me.

I feel a bit sheepish, the current record holder, doing a token lap. Yet, everyone is supportive and assures me of their ongoing prayers. As we cross the starting line again, the runners take off. I walk two more laps for good measure before loving voices encourage me to stop.

"Don't push yourself too hard."

"Don't you have a book to finish?"

So, as they run, I write.

I write with a deep sense that this is what God has for me to do today. I have run before. I pray that I will run again. But for today, I write. And, I remind myself, *Don't let the fact that you can't do what you once did keep you from doing what you can do now.*

I take a break from my typing and wander back to the table at the starting line where the laps are being recorded. The runners are in their third hour. The sun is hot. Drenched bodies pass by with that "this ain't easy" look on their faces. The lead runner is eighty eight laps into his journey. As he passes, he assures me, "Your record is safe again this year."

A spectator asks, "Is this hard for you to watch?"

"Yes," I admit. But I realize that the deep emotions I've felt over the last few years—a list that includes anger, grief, and envy—are quieter now. Healing has come to my soul as well as my body. Not complete healing, but powerful nevertheless.

"I'm praying that you'll run again," a runner announces as he passes by.

I am, too. I'd love to feel strong and free again. I'd love to feel again the wind in my face, stride of my legs, and the renewal of a wooded trail. But more than I desire to run again, I believe I can honestly say that at this point in this mysterious journey, I have two deeper passions: I want to finish well and I long for God to be glorified en route.

Whether I run, walk, or wheelchair my way across the finish line, I want to cross it with my spirit alive and my God exalted. I'm not on the journey I ever expected to be on, I don't have all my questions about it answered, and I don't know where it leads; but if I can be passionate for life all the way to the end and praise my God along the way, I'm convinced that the journey will be good.

Recently, I had the privilege of returning to the gathering of the national conference of our denomination. As I've mentioned, two years earlier the two thousand people in attendance had prayed for me in one of their main services. I didn't feel God's touch upon my body that night, but at their next gathering it was my privilege to speak to the entire assembly. With joy, I reported God's gracious answers to their prayers. I closed my message with an invitation to give God glory. I close this edition of my story with the same invitation.

> Throughout this journey, people have made numerous attempts to explain away what has happened to me. As the nurse removed my feeding tube, I told the story of my swallow being healed. He ignored all references to God and responded, "The body has an amazing way of healing itself."

> As I downed a glass of orange juice, I explained to the friendly guy seated next to me on the airplane that a year ago I couldn't do that. He congratulated me, "You've overcome quite a hurdle."

> As I was getting my haircut, the story of my healing unfolded. Dodging all of my references to God, but curious about my story, the woman cutting my hair cheerfully summarized, "It just goes to show that miracles happen every day!"

> Yes—that's all fine and good: the body is amazing, hurdles can be overcome, and miracles do happen, but don't miss the point! God deserves the glory for this! He's the one who created the body. He's the one who enables us to overcome. He's the source of every miracle!

> I wanted to say to each of these people, "A miracle is sitting next to you and God should get some glory right now!"

In my spirit, I knew it was wrong to give credit to anything or anyone other than God. Praise should be flowing to Jesus. Gratitude should be ascending to God.

The nurse removing my tube won't do it, the guy next to me on the airplane won't do it, the employee at Cost-Cutters won't do it, but will you? Will you give Him glory tonight? Will you thank Him with me?

The congregation stood in praise to God. I stepped off the platform with deep satisfaction. If my story can bring Him glory, I'll keep telling it and I'll keep living it for as many more chapters as He grants me.

Blessings to you as you continue to write your story with Him as well.

# APPENDIX

This book quotes the following songs:

Pg. 48: *A Healing Stream* by Steve Phifer

Pg. 64: *Day By Day* by Andrew L. Skoog, Karolina Wilhelmina Sandell-Berg, and Oskar Ahnfelt

Pg. 65: *He Giveth More Grace* by Annie Johnson Flint and Eric Ashley

Pg. 80: *How Great Is Our God* by Chris Tomlin, Ed Cash, and Jesse Reeves

Pg. 99: *Oh the Deep, Deep Love of Jesus* by Samuel Trevor Francis. Performed by Selah as *Deep, Deep Love* on the "Hiding Place" album.

Pg. 101: *How Great Is Our God* by Chris Tomlin, Ed Cash, and Jesse Reeves

Pg. 101: *God Is In Control* by Twila Paris

Pg. 101: *Don't Let Your Heart Be Hardened* by Bob Hartman

Pg. 102: *You Never Let Go* by Matt Redman

Pg. 113: *There's A River Of Life* by Betty Carr Pulkingham and L. Casebolt

Pg. 172: *I've Got The Victory* by Victor L. Johnson

Pg. 188: *Amazing Grace* by John Newton

Pg. 215: *He Leadeth Me* by Joseph Henry Gilmore

Pg. 222: *I Need Thee Every Hour* by Robert Lowry and Annie Sherwood Hawks

For more information
about John & Joanna,
Nesting Tree Books,
having John speak at your event,
ordering more copies of this book,
or discovering other books that the Stumbos are writing
please visit us at
*johnstumbo.com*